D0306610

Narrative and Stories

Illness, dying, and bereavement

Narrative and Stories in Health Care

Illness, dying, and bereavement

Edited by

Yasmin Gunaratnam

Lecturer, Department of Sociology,
Goldsmiths College,
University of London, UK.

David Oliviere

Director of Education and Training,
St. Christopher's Hospice;
Visiting Professor,
School of Health and Social Sciences,
Middlesex University, UK.

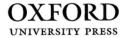

OXFORD
UNIVERSITY PRESS

OXFORD
UNIVERSITY PRESS

Great Clarendon Street, Oxford OX2 6DP

Oxford University Press is a department of the University of Oxford.
It furthers the University's objective of excellence in research, scholarship,
and education by publishing worldwide in

Oxford New York

Auckland Cape Town Dar es Salaam Hong Kong Karachi
Kuala Lumpur Madrid Melbourne Mexico City Nairobi
New Delhi Shanghai Taipei Toronto

With offices in

Argentina Austria Brazil Chile Czech Republic France Greece
Guatemala Hungary Italy Japan Poland Portugal Singapore
South Korea Switzerland Thailand Turkey Ukraine Vietnam

Oxford is a registered trade mark of Oxford University Press
in the UK and in certain other countries

Published in the United States
by Oxford University Press Inc., New York

© Oxford University Press, 2009 (all other chapters)

© Taylor & Francis, 2005 (chapter 9)

The moral rights of the author have been asserted
Database right Oxford University Press (maker)

First published by Oxford University Press 2009

All rights reserved. No part of this publication may be reproduced,
stored in a retrieval system, or transmitted, in any form or by any means,
without the prior permission in writing of Oxford University Press,
or as expressly permitted by law, or under terms agreed with the appropriate
reprographics rights organization. Enquiries concerning reproduction
outside the scope of the above should be sent to the Rights Department,
Oxford University Press, at the address above

You must not circulate this book in any other binding or cover
and you must impose the same condition on any acquirer

British Library Cataloguing in Publication Data

Data available

Library of Congress Cataloging in Publication Data

Data available

Typeset in Minion by Cepha Imaging Private Ltd., Bangalore, India
Printed in Great Britain
on acid-free paper by
The MPG Books Group

ISBN 978–0–19–954669–5 (pbk)

10 9 8 7 6 5 4 3 2 1

Oxford University Press makes no representation, express or implied, that the drug dosages in this
book are correct. Readers must therefore always check the product information and clinical
procedures with the most up-to-date published product information and data sheets provided
by the manufacturers and the most recent codes of conduct and safety regulations. The authors
and the publishers do not accept responsibility or legal liability for any errors in the text or for the
misuse or misapplication of material in this work. Except where otherwise stated, drug dosages and
recommendations are for the non-pregnant adult who is not breast-feeding.

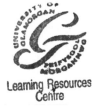

Learning Resources
Centre

13725580

Contents

Contents

Foreword

Barbara Monroe

Several writers in this book remind the reader of Dame Cicely Saunders' use of patient narratives to shame, persuade and finally convince a reluctant health care environment about the need to transform the care of the dying by responding sensitively to the complex needs of patients as individuals within their family and community networks. Along the way the power of that story has sometimes been diluted and even overcome by more powerful narratives. Today health care is once again paying attention to patient and carer stories – user involvement and empowerment is a key part of most end-of-life care strategies, with patient narratives becoming a powerful lobbying tool and 'personalised care' emerging as a significant agenda.

This book is timely, relevant and challenging. It invites us to explore the myriad purposes, meaning and value of stories. Stories help us to find coherence in our lives; to understand our past and to know that despite all obstacles, we can fashion our own future. Stories can help those whose lives have been disrupted by life-threatening illness to grapple with new ways of responding to a hitherto unimaginable future. Listening attentively to individuals can help them to discover a new sense of themselves and the meaning of their lives and develop enhanced confidence and self-respect. When we bring dying individuals together, either in groups or simply by sharing the experiences of others, we begin to offer them alternative possibilities, new versions of the future. Good care helps to remind people that whatever the pain of what is happening now, it should not and cannot engulf the rest of their lives. It is one chapter among many and individuals can still choose to be author of their futures. My personal encounters with dying people and those close to them have convinced me, like many clinicians, that stories can become vehicles for truth and that such truths can carry healing.

This book does not ignore the problems of narrative work, nor the importance of the ethics surrounding it. Arthur Frank memorably outlines the 'trickster' dangers that constantly lie in wait in the use of narrative in end-of-life care. Stories are not always benevolent in their impact and our hearing can be sadly unidimensional. He describes how coercive other people's dominant narratives can be: for example, explicit or implicit exhortations to see illness as a 'battle' or to be grateful for the 'benefits' it conveys. Frank also notes the power of institutional narratives to silence or distort individual goals. Gail Eva emphasizes how professional assessments of patient stories and their reliability can affect access to services. Set against these caveats are magnificent examples of the power of stories to create new possibilities. Patsy Way describes work with bereaved children and their families where stories are used to break the silence that so often descends and to suggest new ways of remembering the past and alternative identities for the future. Jonathan Koffman's thoughtful analysis of his own research efforts demonstrates how sensitive listening can generate new understandings about the complex meanings individuals attribute to illness and symptoms.

The value of narrative work is not limited to the patient. Gunaratnam and Oliviere's well-organized volume begins with an examination of the theoretical concepts of narrative and story and the value of narrative-based evidence and research. It then explores the role of narrative in influencing service development and finally the power of storytelling and making in direct clinical work. The book also demonstrates the value of stories in the training of health care professionals and in campaigning and advocacy.

The experience of life-threatening illness or bereavement can leave us bewildered, confused, and isolated: alone with fragments that make no sense. Telling the story to someone who listens carefully and without prejudice can both heal and help the hurt individual to find a new sense of meaning, purpose, and control. This book is a comprehensive guide to the issues and the possibilities of narrative and stories in end-of-life care.

Acknowledgements

Heart-felt thanks to the contributors to this collection, who showed great trust in us from the outset and who produced essays that far exceeded our expectations. We have learned so much not only about narrative and stories through their scholarship, but also about generosity and care. The idea for the book was inspired by a study day at St Christopher's Hospice in 2007 and the contributions of participants helped us to frame our initial ideas and thinking about the demands and possibilities of a narrative-based palliative care. We are particularly grateful to Georgia Pinteau at Oxford University Press, who with Eloise Moir Ford, encouraged and supported us in the early stages of the manuscript and to Helen Hill and Gayathri Bellan who steered and managed the production process. The book would not have been possible without the support, insight and suggestions of the anonymous reviewers. Alida Gersie, Prue Chamberlayne and Tom Wengraf challenged and sharpened our thinking about narrative and story-telling. Special thanks to our families and colleagues for their continued support and patience.

List of contributors

Gillie Bolton
Freelance Consultant and
Writer: medical humanities,
reflective practice writing,
therapeutic writing, UK

Phil Cotterell
Senior Research Fellow,
Macmillan Research Unit,
School of Health Sciences,
University of Southampton, UK;
Formerly Research Fellow,
Health and Social Policy
Research Centre,
University of Brighton, UK

Sayantani DasGupta
Assistant Professor of
Clinical Pediatrics, Division
of General Pediatrics and Core
Faculty Member, Program in
Narrative Medicine, Columbia
University, USA

Kim Devery
Acting Head of Department,
Department of Palliative and
Supportive Services, Flinders
University Adelaide, Australia

Gail Eva
Research Fellow,
Nuffield Department of Clinical
Medicine, and Harris Manchester
College University of Oxford, UK
Senior Lecturer in Palliative Care,
Oxford Brookes University, UK

Helen Findlay
Communications Consultant
working in the charitable, voluntary
and local government sectors, UK

Karen Forbes
Consultant and Macmillan
Professorial Teaching Fellow,
Department of Palliative
Medicine, Bristol Haematology
and Oncology Centre, UK

Arthur Frank
Professor of Sociology,
University of Calgary, Canada

Yasmin Gunaratnam
Lecturer, Department of Sociology,
Goldsmiths College,
University of London, UK

Craig Irvine
Assistant Professor, Center for
Family and Community Medicine,
and Core Faculty Member,
Program in Narrative Medicine,
Columbia University, USA

Jonathan Koffman
Lecturer in Palliative Care,
King's College London School of
Medicine, UK

William Alwyn Lishman
Emeritus Professor of
Neuropsychiatry, Institute of
Psychiatry,
London, UK

Ann Macfarlane MBE
Consultant in Disability
Equality, Rights and
Independent Living, UK

Barbara Monroe
Chief Executive, St Christopher's
Hospice, UK

David Oliviere
Director of Education and Training,
St Christopher's Hospice;
Visiting Professor, School of
Health and Social Sciences,
Middlesex University, UK

John Paley
Senior Lecturer, Department of
Nursing and Midwifery,
University of Stirling,
Scotland, UK

Irene Renzenbrink
Educator and Consultant in
Palliative Care and Bereavement
Support, Australia

Maura Spiegel
Senior Lecturer, Department of
English and Comparative Literature,
and Core Faculty Member
Program in Narrative Medicine,
Columbia University, USA;
Term Professor;
Barnard College, USA

Rachel Stanworth
Lecturer Practitioner in
Palliative Care,
Compton Hospice,
Wolverhampton, UK

Tony Walter
Professor of Death Studies,
Centre for Death and Society,
University of Bath, UK

Patsy Way
Family Therapist and
Project Worker, Candle Project,
St Christopher's Hospice, UK

Introduction

Yasmin Gunaratnam and David Oliviere

Irene, a patient at a London cancer hospital, took just six minutes to tell her story, with ruminations on care, treatment, death, and bereavement. She began with 'This is a wonderful place . . . they have a cure for everything' and ended with 'They are just going to get me through to Christmas . . . and then decide what to do with me. I'm worried about Bill looking after himself'.

Clinically and therapeutically, stories and narratives are integral to the provision of care. As a form of expression, stories can draw near to the interconnected holism of experience (Polkinghorne, 1988), a point recognized by D.H. Lawrence when he wrote, 'The novel is the highest form of subtle interrelatedness that man has discovered' (quoted in Leavis, 1967: 11). A story conveys information about events, and emotion and *knowledge*; it can affect the listener/reader and a situation; and it allows us to *acknowledge* the person and affirm their narrated experience (Frank, 2000). In health and social care, it has been argued that narratives and stories have specific significance (Frank, 1995; Froggett, 2002; Mattingly, 1998). Those who are ill can use narrative to make sense of the 'biographical disruption' (Bury, 1982) and losses of illness (Williams, 1984), and professional narratives can function to maintain identity (McDermott et al. 2006), and as fora for imaginative projections (Becker, 2005) and ethical deliberation (Gunaratnam, 2008).

This concern with the workings and the effects of narratives and stories is central to this collection of essays. In their contributions, authors – many of whom are recognized as leading experts in their fields – demonstrate and reflect upon the use and value, but also the unsubstantiated claims and shortcomings of narrative approaches in palliative and end-of-life care.

As an entry into narrative work with people who are ill and dying, we turn to questions of shared meaning, language, and terminology that are the basis of active participation in both dialogue and community. For the purposes of this book, we recognize that narrative approaches encompass a range of media, from the written and the spoken, to rituals and art (Romanoff and Thompson, 2006). The distinction between a 'story' and a 'narrative' is also significant, and we have drawn from the work of John Paley and Gail Eva (2005) who offer the following definitions: a story involves 'an interweaving of plot and character, whose organization is designed to elicit a certain emotional response . . . while "narrative" refers to the sequence of events and the (claimed) causal connections between them' (p. 83). In this sense 'narrative' is a common denominator: all stories are narratives, but not all narratives have the organizational structure or evoke the emotional reaction of stories (Paley and Eva, 2005).

The distinction between narratives and stories is not simply linguistic and conceptual and marks the use of the terms as work in the caring professions. At a broad level, the academic literature tends to address and engage with 'narrative', while practitioners, particularly those working with psycho-dynamic and artistic methods, refer to 'stories' and 'storytelling'; a difference and tension that is related, undoubtedly, to divisions between 'objective' and 'subjective' approaches to human experience and which open up questions about ways of knowing, relating, and working.

Such questions underpin the contributions that follow and relate to our concern about the development of narrative work as a craft involving the use of skills, tools and judgement, a connecting of hand and head, and a desire to a do a job well (Sennett, 2008). Using the scholarship of the political philosopher Hannah Arendt (1958/1998), Sennett identifies two predominant images in modern thinking of people at work: *Animal laborens*, ground down with demanding routines and tasks that block out the wider world, and *Homo faber* who stops and thinks and talks with others about the purpose of the work once it is completed. For Arendt, it was this reflecting and talking that was the foundation of ethics, but as thinking-after-doing it is in a sense always too late and Sennett suggests that a more balanced view would be recognizing that 'thinking and feeling are contained within the process of making' (p. 7). Sennett holds that:

> Every good craftsman conducts a dialogue between concrete practices and thinking; this dialogue evolves into sustaining habits, and these habits establish a rhythm between problem solving and problem finding. The relation between hand and head appears in domains seemingly as different as bricklaying, cooking, designing and playground, or playing the cello – but all these practices can misfire or fail to ripen. There is nothing inevitable about becoming skilled, just as there is nothing mindlessly mechanical about technique itself. (p. 9)

Most of us will know exactly what Richard Sennett is describing here and a hope for this book is that it might contribute to a 'rhythm' of narrative work that is simultaneously affirming and questioning, and that provokes dialogue and critical reflection.

Narrative and palliative care

As some readers may be aware, narrative and stories are a part of the creation myth of modern hospice and palliative care. Organizational creation myths have been seen not so much in terms of fabrication and fiction, but as providing a symbolic ordering to institutional life that 'helps to configure a system of meaning and a collective imaginary' (Froggett and Chamberlayne, 2004: 63). The creation myth of modern hospice care began over half a century ago with Cicely Saunders – regarded as the founder of the modern hospice movement. At this time, Saunders was working among dying people in London, collecting their stories of illness and pain and pioneering a methodology of alchemy: turning patient narratives and stories into a philosophy and practice of holistic care for dying people.

For Saunders, narrative methods held an opportunity to practise medicine in a way that facilitated meaningful connections with patients, through which she was able to transpose the singularity of their experiences into the work of clinical practice. Insights into this approach can be found in a talk Saunders gave to a London hospital in 1961:

> I am fortunate too, above all, in being a doctor who isn't in a hurry, so that I have time to know and to enjoy my patients, and I very often take a portable tape-recorder round with me, which, of course, they all know about. It is a very great help, both to get permanent records of them talking about their pain and its relief, but also about their attitudes towards their illness; what they know about it, and what they find particularly hard, and it is very revealing, both for them, and about myself too when I play it back.
>
> (quoted in Clark[1], 1999: 729)

Cicely Saunders recorded over 1000 patient narratives and attributed these accounts to the development of basic concepts in palliative care such as 'total pain' which recognizes the multiple sources and interventions needed to resolve the physical, psychological, social, emotional, and spiritual aspects of pain (Saunders, 1979).

From its very beginnings then, modern palliative care has always involved a variety of forms of care. It can include the bespoke calculation of pain control medication, physiotherapy, and rehabilitation, support with accessing welfare benefits, and the counselling of patients and those close to them. These types of practice differ in their empirical content and in the theories of knowledge (epistemology) that inform them, yet each area of work, as in medicine more generally, will at some point in time be 'indelibly stamped with the telling or receiving or creating of stories' (Charon, 2006: vii). Karen Forbes (Chapter 7) writes that 'Healthcare is a storied world', and as Bingley et al. (2008: 653) observe, 'The telling of stories has been a vital currency of reporting the experience of end of life care over the last 50 years'. Yet it has not always been so, and many writers have pointed to how the significance given to techniques and practices that attempt to access patients' subjective experiences of illness have sprung from the demands of historically shifting regimes of medical knowledge and power (Armstrong, 1983; Foucault, 1976).

As she herself recognized, Cicely Saunders's work was very much of its time, being given impetus through a series of developments during the 1950s and 1960s, including the introduction of psychotropic drugs, surveys, and reports on patient need, pain clinics, and psychoanalytic work on loss and bereavement (Saunders, 1988). This wave of change also involved what is now commonly referred to as the 'turn to narrative' (see Chamberlayne et al. 2000). In health care, this 'turn' has been connected to critiques of medical dominance and models of health and illness made by sociologists and anthropologists; changes in morbidity patterns with a higher incidence of people 'living with' diseases such as cancer (so that patients' accounts of their illness are central to care management); the expansion of patient information and 'illness narratives'; and the development of patient or 'user' participation as a part of 'new social movements' (Bury, 2001).

Despite incursions by bureaucratic and market-driven imperatives (James and Field, 1992), the value of using narratives and stories to engage with personal realities and perspectives, for patients, carers, and professionals, is being given increased attention in the palliative care literature (Barnard et al. 2000; Bingley et al. 2006; Brown, 2008; Brown and Addington-Hall, 2007; Gunaratnam, 2004; Hallenbeck, 2003; McDermott et al. 2006; Romanoff and Thompson, 2006; Stanworth, 2004). This literature has emphasized the potential for narrative to create and express meaning, to mediate painful and difficult experiences, and to encapsulate the complicated relationships between the individual and their social and material circumstances.

As Arthur Frank (Chapter 10) observes, 'Stories and storytelling are popular these days; narrative is in vogue'; nonetheless, as we will make clear, although this popularity has much to offer, we also need to be alert to the potential limitations and dangers of our approaches and work with narrative and stories.

Narrative dangers

In many ways it is the ubiquity and the very ordinariness of narrative that is both a strength and a disadvantage in palliative care, where the multidisciplinary foundations of the discipline hold what some have seen as the deep tensions that exist in medicine between objective and subjective forms of knowledge and between anatomical and psycho-social realities (Hawthorne and Yurkovich, 2003; Hurwitz et al. 2004). Consider, for example, one particularly helpful and honest review of the proposal for this book in which the reviewer wrote:

> Would I buy this book or use it? As a clinician with a fair understanding of research probably not, mainly because time is precious and I'm not sure of the creditworthiness etc of this type of research. I would have to be sure of its practical application. As an academic/lecturer I could see how this could be used as a teaching resource and I would like to gain more of an insight into the claims of narrative

Such ambivalence towards narrative, scepticism about its 'creditworthiness', and the suggestion of disciplinary divisions in palliative care with regard to questions about its 'practical application' are not uncommon and need to be given careful thought and consideration. Rather than seeking to counter such ambivalence and doubt with a proselytizing about the inherent power of narrative and stories, the chapters in this collection take a different approach. Our starting point is the day-to-day work of care for ill and dying people – in all of its variations and sites. From this starting point we recognize that the 'turn to narrative' has contributed, and continues to contribute, much to the validation of patient experiences (Frank, 1995; Kleinman, 1988), and to clinical and psycho-social care, for example, through 'narrative-based medicine' (Charon, 2006; Greenhalgh and Hurwitz, 1998) and 'narrative therapy' (Charles-Edwards, 2007). Nevertheless, as several contributors to this volume suggest, there is also need for a critical examination of narrative work, so that we have a fuller sense of both what narrative can offer, as well as its constraints and 'dangers'.

The three introductory chapters to each section of the book take up this theme of the potency and constraints of narrative in different ways. John Paley (Chapter 1) provides a provocative and forensic examination of the conceptual distinctions between narrative and story, demonstrating through a spectrum of examples from jokes to illness narratives, how the different structural components of a story can function together to produce its impact. Paley's discussion shows the common confusions and lazy assumptions that are a part of narrative work, while also engaging with the pithy ethical question of when, and in what circumstances, 'believing seductive falsehoods, may be rationally and ethically acceptable'.

Gail Eva (Chapter 6) animates and applies concepts from literary criticism regarding the meaning, performance, and effect of stories to her empirical research in evaluating the provision of hospice rehabilitation to patients with metastatic spinal cord compression. Through a close-up reading of the stories of two different patients, and staff responses to these stories, Eva's analysis makes clear *how* the structuring of a patient's story works to cast them as either reliable or unreliable narrators, thereby affecting professional assessments of their needs and determining the patient's access to a service. A significant challenge that Eva identifies is how palliative care professionals might respect patients' self-presentation, while also 'nudging' them towards behaviours that support their well-being.

In the 'The necessity and dangers of illness narratives' (Chapter 10), Arthur Frank builds upon his ground-breaking work in *The Wounded Storyteller* (1995) in which he both advocated the importance of storytelling for those who are ill, and examined the healing power and moral qualities of illness narratives. His most recent reflections find him exploring 'a darker side' of storytelling, an area which he recognizes as being underdeveloped in his previous scholarship. Using the trope of the 'trickster' Frank identifies four dangers of stories as they relate to: narrative form, genre problems, coercive potential, and moral insularity. Echoing the challenges for professional practice and care identified in Eva's chapter, Frank suggests that 'The delicate balance of clinical work is how gently or how hard to push people off one story and towards another.'

A 'blank cry'

Our engagement with the potential dangers of narrative is not so much a 'turn against narrative' as an exploration of what happens when narrative comes up against its limits, for instance in situations of pain and suffering (Bar-On, 1999; Scarry, 1985), and ultimately in death. In Chapter 2, Practitioners from the Program in Narrative Medicine at Colombia University recount the experiences of a student doctor Ashley, who in the midst of 5 hours of intense medical intervention to prevent a patient's respiratory decline, was assigned to hold the patient's hand. The patient died and Ashley felt 'helpless' and 'useless', only writing and talking about the trauma of this experience two years later, during Craig Irvine's elective narrative ethics course. The authors suggest that narrating the experience was a way in which Ashley could come to recognize the role that she played in accompanying the patient sensually and emotionally to her death. Yet, this example also speaks of the limits of narrative at times of suffering and death, and the value, but also the profound difficulty of receptiveness and passivity as care (DasGupta, 2007; Gunaratnam, 2008; Hoggett, 2000; Waddell, 1989).

There are times when narrative is exceeded, is itself 'helpless' and 'useless', and we need to interrogate as our reviewer did, its 'practical application', and also any assumptions we might have about a universal 'narritavising core' (Frosh, 2007: 635) that lies at the heart of all human experiences (see Lieblich et al. 1998). Might our recourse to claims about the transcendental and restorative powers of narrative at times of illness, its capacity to 'mend the things that are broken' (Bausch, 2001), sometimes function as a personal and organizational 'defence mechanism' (Menzies Lyth, 1988) in palliative care, helping us to avoid or deny painful and unfathomable events, or perhaps to speak as 'artificial persons' (Frank, 2004) who mouth official discourses that sideline professional vulnerability? This is a sensitive and difficult area to discuss, not only for those who work with narrative and stories and have witnessed their value, but also because it challenges deeply held Western beliefs about human capability as being realized through activity (Derrida, 2002; Levinas, 1978).

There are many reasons as to why clinicians (among others) should be sceptical about the claims made about narrative. We would like to think that some of this scepticism arises not solely from antagonism to the different and more ambiguous ways of knowing advocated by narrative epistemologies (Lieblich et al. 1998), but from the fleshy realities of daily work with ill and dying people. It is a profound paradox that in the very midst of the intensity of human relations that surround dying and death, there is the non-relational and what Clark refers to as 'an irreducible facticity' (1993: 3) – bodily processes and states that mark a withdrawal from word and world. It is such processes that the Russian poet Anna Akhmatova (1985: 45) evoked when she wrote, 'Wild honey has the scent of freedom/ dust of a ray of sun/ a girl's mouth – of a violet ... but we have found out forever/ that blood smells only of blood'.

'The nonrelational is that which offers no purchase' Harrison writes, 'which eludes in a passivity which if it may be said to resist at all has the inert resistance of a weakness beyond or outside power, like a "blank cry"' (2007: 593). Receptivity to the demands of this 'blank cry' (Chretien, 2004: 6) entails recognition of how narrative can fail and fall short in the face of human suffering and at times of death. As much as narrative is able to create new social and personal realities, as much as it is machinery that 'does things' (see Frank, 2006, and Paley, this volume), it can also become exhausted and superfluous in the falling away of the body and personhood in dying. Here, there seems great value in pursuing further discussion about what lies outside of narrative at such times, what emerges from its incapacity, and what this means for how we understand and practise care.

The book

An exploration of narrative work in palliative and end-of-life care – what it can, and cannot do, and how we might work with narrative methods – is much needed. Despite the longevity and the renewal of interest in narratives and storytelling in the specialty, the literature, and the knowledge and experiences of those who use the methods are diverse and fragmented. There are inconsistencies in the use of the basic terms 'narrative' and 'story' and in the respective assumptions that are made about them, prompting some authors to call for 'narrative vigilance' (Paley and Eva, 2005). Such inconsistencies cannot be separated from the diversity in methodological approaches to narrative or the significant gaps that exist between academic approaches and the use of narratives and storytelling among practitioners.

In what follows we aim to both elucidate and lessen this fragmentation of knowledge and practice by bringing into closer dialogue the worlds of theory and practice. The book will address and clarify key issues: What is a narrative? What is a story? What are some of the main methods and models that can be used in palliative care, and for what purposes? What are their respective strengths and weaknesses? What practical and ethical dilemmas can the methods entail? How can we use narratives and stories to enhance care?

The book is divided into three distinct, but interrelated parts. Section one provides an introduction to narratives and stories in research, as 'evidence' and in professional practice in palliative care. The second section focuses upon how narratives and stories have been used in service development. And section three consists of chapters that examine narrative and stories in work with patients and carers and in clinical and psycho-social care. The opening chapter for each of the three sections is what we have envisaged as a scene-setting chapter. These foundational chapters aim to introduce the reader to key concepts, debates, and themes that relate to the broad subject matter of each section.

Section 1 begins with John Paley's wide-ranging discussion of 'Narrative machinery', examining and clarifying concepts, and investigating how the machinery of narrative works, why it is used and what its use can achieve. Paley marks the distinction between narrative and story through the 'teleogenic plot' with culminates in denouement. It is Paley's contention that 'the story threshold is the point at which narrative acquires a teleogenic plot'. The chapters that follow in this section provide a variety of settings in which Paley's ideas and claims can be applied and further examined.

Writing from the Program in Narrative Medicine at Colombia, DasGupta, Irvine, and Spiegel begin by addressing the potential fruitfulness of the inter-relations between palliative care and narrative medicine. They ask 'what can narrative medicine offer palliative care?' and sketch out what 'a narratively based palliative care' might look like: reflexive, relationship rather than technique based, and characterized by the 'attention, representation and affiliation' of Charon's (2006) 'narrative competence'. Gunaratnam explores related themes in her chapter on narrative research. Drawing upon a single case-study – a method commonly used in biographical narrative research – Gunaratnam details the principles and the assumptions that underlie narrative interviews and that can also be used in clinical practice, where she sees the narrative practitioner as a midwife to narrative, helping and coaxing narrative into the world. Through her interviewing relationship with a hospice patient 'Phyllis', Gunaratnam reflects upon the ethics of narrative incoherence and irresolution in interpretation, where a concern with the craftwork of methodology includes being 'faithful to the unknown'.

Kim Devery (Chapter 4) takes the focus upon narrative and research in a different direction, considering how narrative might contribute to the evidence base in palliative care. Devery's forceful argument is that palliative care's commitment to holistic, person-centre care demands multiple sources of evidence, but also dialogue that moves towards 'a collective story for the discipline that connected and contextualized different professional beliefs, morals and expectations'. While staying with research, Gillie Bolton takes us to the bedside and the wards of teenage cancer patients, drawing upon the findings of an exploratory study that she participated in on the use and value of therapeutic creative writing in oncology settings. Bolton's study found that creative writing can be cathartic and can enhance self-respect and confidence, mapping the past and helping young people to orientate to the future. As one participant in Bolton's research wrote, 'Writing is a way of saying things I can't say. I do it when I'm on my own, and as a way of coping with being down'.

In Section 2 of the book, the focus is very much upon narratives and stories in service provision. Here, contrasting chapters tackle what many would see as the 'practical' implications of narrative work in the everyday delivery of care services. Eva's chapter demonstrates the importance not only of good listening, but also of critical analysis in interpreting the meaning and effects of patient and professional narratives (see above). Karen Forbes (Chapter 7) introduces readers to a range of approaches to the use of narrative in teaching and learning, including history taking, reflective practice, action research, and appreciative inquiry. In a powerful case-study drawn from her teaching, Forbes shows how narrative can be used to teach medical students about working closely with death and dying. Many students become distressed during such teaching and Forbes describes how 'each time the room is completely silent, each time I look up briefly and scan faces, each time I see tears'. Yet her argument is that despite the risks involved, the emotion-rich content of narrative can enable students to recognize, in a safe environment, the compassion and humanity that will be demanded of them as doctors.

The realities of patient and carer experiences are brought home in Cotterell, Findlay and Macfarlane's chapter. The chapter considers narrative and stories in the broader context of 'user involvement' in palliative care. Helen Findlay writes of her family's distressing experiences of caring for her father as he died of Motor Neurone Disease (MND) in a general hospital. Determined to improve the end of life care of other people with MND, Findlay documents the work of her family in recording their experiences in the 'Findlay Report' and then employing 'guerrilla tactics' to disseminate the report and its recommendations. Ann Macfarlane charts her varying experiences of hospice care as a disabled person and shows how a superficial engagement with narratives of 'independence' can be physically and emotionally damaging for disabled people who use hospice services. While recognizing the emotional effects of narrative, the authors suggest that such emotionality is an inescapable part of care experiences which need to be acknowledged and attended to.

Tony Walter's chapter on 'Mediator Deathwork' looks at the production of narrative accounts and stories from professionals working outside of the framework of traditional professional–patient relationships. Drawing upon innovative research with these 'mediator death workers' who include pathologists, coroners, clergy, and funeral celebrants, Walter describes how these professionals work with 'private' information about the dead person and use this information to produce stories that become a part of a more public story and record. By uncovering this much neglected area of work, the chapter demonstrates how mediator death work can be a significant part of the care for bereaved people, warranting far greater recognition and attention.

The focus in Section 3 of the book is on patients and carers. The introductory chapter by Frank (see above) makes explicit how narrative can work to situate and connect principles with practical action for both patients and professionals, particularly at the end of life. Frank advocates clinical commitment to support three aspects of individuals' storytelling as they relate to: the choices that people make about the stories in their lives; how they interpret these stories; and their responsibility for thinking about the effects of their stories. Renzenbrink develops the theme of narrative as care in her examination of life story and life review work that describes practical methods and models that have been used in different disciplinary settings and cultural contexts including England, New Zealand, and Canada. The chapter draws particular attention to the emotional challenges of such work, the need for staff to receive training, supervision, and support, and the need to remain cautious about the increasing technology surrounding reminiscence work at the end of life.

Using qualitative research, Koffman's chapter (Chapter 12) investigates the common and differing meanings of pain and symptoms in the narratives of White British and Black Caribbean patients with advanced cancer. During his research Koffman made efforts to suspend his expectations about what illness and dying might mean to his research participants; to his surprise he found how for some Black Caribbean patients cancer was not the most challenging experience they had lived through, while others talked about welcoming death as it connected them more closely with god. Koffman's work reiterates the importance of attention to patients' narratives in producing a more complete picture of clinical problems and in recognizing how social difference can affect narrative form and content.

Rachel Stanworth's chapter (Chapter 13) on spirituality defined as 'the interpretive story and values of shared human experience', combines a deft interweaving of insights from theological and philosophical literature, with examples from her ongoing work in palliative care. While acknowledging the value of narrative analysis, Stanworth brings us to the mysteries and poetics of narrated experience as they are disclosed through symbol, metaphor, and paradox and which demand 'committed attention'. Such attentiveness can be seen in Patsy Way's description and discussion of her therapeutic work as a part of the Candle Project at St Christopher's Hospice that provides bereavement care to children (Chapter 14). Way introduces us to the stories of Patrick and his companion 'Mr Trouble'; Shiv and his struggles with grief and a new family positioning; Gemma and the 'wicked stepmother' story; and Jude and Ali whose fathers died when they were very young. For Way, therapeutic work with narrative 'can allow twists and alternative possibilities in real lives. Twists and possibilities that it might be hard to think about and reach in other ways'.

In the 'Afterword', Alwyn Lishman draws upon his professional expertise in psychiatry and his experiences of user-involvement initiatives as a former carer, where he noticed that telling stories was vital to facilitating patients' and carers' participation in meetings and committees. Recognizing the breadth of narrative work in palliative care, Lishman identifies and homes in on a singular contribution of narrative and storytelling to care – 'placing the individual at the centre of the picture'.

Endings and new places

Mishler (1999) has depicted the work of prefacing and introducing a book as 'a place of exits and entrances' (p. vii); a place that marks a series of emotional and intellectual encounters, with authors leaving their work behind them, and readers entering into, and wandering through the spaces of what is left behind. We hope that what you find will be of value and that you might take it to new and surprising places.

Notes

1. This excerpt is from a talk entitled: 'I was sick and you visited me', given at St Mary's Hospital, London, 30 May 1961; Cicely Saunders' archive, St Christopher's Hospice, Sydenham.

References

Akhmatova, A. (1985) *Twenty Poems – Anna Akhmatova*. Trans Jane Keyon, Eighties Press and Ally Press, Minnesota.

Arendt, H. (1998) *The Human Condition* (2nd edn). University of Chicago Press, Chicago.

Armstrong, D. (1983) *Political Anatomy of the Body: Medical Knowledge in Britain in the Twentieth Century*. Cambridge University Press, Cambridge.

Barnard, D., Towers, A., Boston, P., and Lambrinidou, Y. (2000) *Crossing Over: Narratives of Palliative Care*. Oxford University Press, New York.

Bar-On, D. (1999) *The Indescribable and the Undiscussable: Reconstructing Human Discourse after Trauma*. Central European University Press, Budapest.

Bausch, C. (2001) The healing story of loss and grief. Congress of the European Association for Palliative care, Palermo.

Becker R (2005) Short stories (editorial). *International Journal of Palliative Nursing*, **11**(2), 52.

Bingley, A. F., McDermott, E., Thomas, C., Payne, S., Seymour, J., and Clark, D. (2006) Making sense of dying: a review of narratives written since 1950 by people facing death from cancer and other diseases. *Palliative Medicine*, **20**(3), 183–95.

Bingley, A., Thomas, C., Brown, J., Reeves, J., and Payne, S. (2008) Developing narrative research in supportive and palliative care: the focus on illness narratives. *Palliative Medicine*, **22**(5), 653–58.

Brown, J. (2008) The need for narrative research. *End of Life Care*, **2**(3), 62–63.

Brown, J. and Addington-Hall, J. (2007) How people with motor neurone disease talk about living with their illness: a narrative study. *Journal of Advanced Nursing*, **62**(2), 200–08.

Bury, M. (1982) Chronic illness as biographical disruption. *Sociology of Health and Illness*, **4**(2), 167–82.

Bury, M. (2001) Illness narratives: fact or fiction? *Sociology of Health and Illness*, **23**(3), 263–85.

Charon, R. (2006) *Narrative Medicine: Honoring the Stories of Illness*. Oxford University Press, Oxford and New York.

Chamberlayne, P., Bornat, J., and Wengraf, T. (eds) (2000) *The Turn to Biographical Methods in Social Science: Comparative Issues and Examples*. Routledge, London.

Clark, D. (1993) Introduction. In *The Sociology of Death* (ed. D. Clark). Blackwell Publishers/The Sociological Review, Oxford, pp. 1–30.

Clark, D. (1999) 'Total pain', disciplinary power and the body in the work of Cicely Saunders, 1958–1967, *Social Science and Medicine*, **49**, 727–36.

Charles-Edwards, D. (2007) Neimeyer and the construction of loss. *Therapy Today*. **18**(5), 15–17.

Chretien, J.-L. (2004) *The Call and the Response*. Fordham University Press, New York.

DasGupta, S. (2007) Between stillness and story: lessons of children's illness narratives. *Pediatrics*, **119**(6), 1384–91.

Derrida, J. (2002) *Without Alibi*. Stanford University Press, Stanford, CA.

Foucault, M. (1976) *The Birth of the Clinic*, Tavistock, London.

Frank, A. (1995) *The Wounded Storyteller: Body, Illness and Ethics*. University of Chicago Press, Chicago, IL.

Frank, A. (2000) Illness and autobiographical work: dialogue as narrative destabilization. *Qualitative Sociology*, **23**(1), 135–56.

Frank, A. (2004) *The Renewal of Generosity: Illness, Medicine, and How to Live*. University of Chicago Press, Chicago, IL.

Frank, A. (2006) Health stories as connectors and subjectifiers. *Health: An Interdisciplinary Journal for the Social Study of Health, Illness, and Medicine*, **10**(4), 421–40.

Froggett, L. (2002) *Love, Hate and Welfare: Psychosocial Approaches to Policy and Practice*. Policy Press, Bristol.

Froggett, L. and Chamberlayne, P. (2004) From biography to practice and policy critique: a case study of community innovation. *Qualitative Social Work*, **3**(1), 55–70.

Frosh, S. (2007) Disintegrating qualitative research. *Theory and Psychology*, **17**, 635–53.

Greenhalgh, T. and Hurwitz, B. (1998) *Narrative Based Medicine: Dialogue and Discourse in Clinical Practice*. BMJ Books, London.

Gunaratnam, Y. (2004) 'Bucking and kicking': 'race', gender and embodied resistance in health care. In *Biographical Methods and Professional Practice: An International Perspective* (eds. U. Apitzsch, J. Bornat, and P. Chamberlayne). Policy Press, Bristol. pp. 205–19.

Gunaratnam, Y. (2008) From competence to vulnerability: care, ethics and elders from racialised minorities. *Mortality*, **13**(1), 24–41.

Hallenbeck, J. (2003) *A Narrative Handbook in Palliative Care: Palliative Care Perspectives*. Oxford University Press, New York.

Harrison, P. (2007) "How shall I say it …?" Relating the nonrelational. *Environment and Planning* A, **39**, 590–608.

Hawthorne, R.N. and Yurkovich, N. (2003) Human relationship: The forgotten dynamic in palliative care. *Palliative & Supportive Care*, **1**, 261–65.

Hoggett, P. (2000) *Emotional Life and the Politics of Welfare*. Basingstoke: Macmillan.

Hurwitz, B., Greenhalgh, T., and Skultans, V. (2004) Introduction. In *Narrative Research in Health and Illness* (eds. B. Hurwitz, T. Greenhalgh, and V. Skultans). BMJ Books, London. pp. 1–20.

James, N. and Field, D. (1992). The routinization of hospice: charisma and bureaucratization. *Social Science and Medicine*, **34**(12), 1363–75.

Kleinman, A. (1988) *The Illness Narratives: Suffering, Healing and the Human Condition*. Basic Books, New York.

Leavis, F.R. (1967) *Anna Karenina and Other Essays*, Chatto and Windus, London.

Levinas, E. (1978) *Existence and Existents*, Kluwer, London.

Lieblich, A., Tuval-Mashiach, R., and Zilber, T. (1998) *Narrative Research: Reading, Analysis and Interpretation*. Sage, London.

Mattingly, C. (1998) *Healing Dramas and Clinical Plots: The Narrative Structure of Experience*, Cambridge University Press, Cambridge.

McDermott, E., Bingley, A.F., Thomas, C., Payne, S., Seymour, J., and Clark, D. (2006) Viewing patient need through professional writings: a systematic 'ethnographic' review of palliative care professionals' experiences of caring for people with cancer at the end of life. *Progress in Palliative Care*, **14**(1), 9–18.

Menzies-Lyth, I. (1988) Containing anxiety in institutions, selected essays. Free Association Books, London.

Mishler, E. (1999) *Storylines: Craftartists' Narratives of Identity*. Harvard University Press, Cambridge, MA and London.

Paley, J. and Eva, G. (2005) Narrative vigilance: the analysis of stories in health care. *Nursing Philosophy*, **6**, 83–97.

Polkinghorne, D. (1988) *Narrative Knowing and the Human Sciences*. State University of New York Press, Albany, NY.

Romanoff, B. and Thompson, B. (2006) Meaning construction in palliative care: the use of narrative, ritual, and the expressive arts. *American Journal of Hospice and Palliative Care*, **23**, 309–16.

Saunders, C. (1979) *The Management of Terminal Disease*. Edward Arnold, London.

Saunders C. (1988) The evolution of the hospices. In *The History of Pain Management: From Early Principles to Present Practice* (ed. R. Mann). Parthenon, Carnforth, pp. 167–78.

Scarry, E. (1985) *The Body in Pain – The Making and Unmaking of the World*. Oxford University Press, New York and Oxford.

Sennett, R. (2008) *The Craftsman*. Allen Lane, Penguin Books, London.

Stanworth, R. (2004) *Recognising Spiritual Needs in People Who Are Dying*. Oxford University Press, Oxford.

Waddell, M. (1989) Living in two worlds: psychodynamic theory and social work practice. *Free Associations*, **15**, 11–35.

Williams, G. (1984) The genesis of chronic illness: narrative reconstruction. *Sociology of Health and Illness*, **6**(2), 175–200.

Section 1

Concepts and approaches

Chapter 1

Narrative machinery

John Paley

Sherlock Holmes and Doctor Watson go on a camping trip. At 2:00 in the morning Holmes wakes his companion, who has been in a deep sleep: 'Look up at the sky, Watson, and tell me what you see.' 'I see stars, Holmes. It is a wonderfully clear night, and I see a million beautiful stars.' 'Excellent', replies Holmes. 'And what, pray, do you deduce from this?' Watson ponders for a moment. 'That the universe is immense, awe-inspiring and sublime, and that we are completely insignificant in comparison?' 'No', says Holmes curtly. 'Somebody's stolen our tent.'

Jokes, which represent just one category in the classification 'story', strip that classification down to its barest form and illustrate, economically, the structure which makes stories what they are, the narrative machinery that makes them work. It is this machinery that I will be examining in this chapter: how it is configured, why it is deployed, what it is intended to produce. To those who are nervous about the metaphor I can, unfortunately, offer no apology. Like machines, stories are ways of getting things done. They process raw material, they generate output, they are efficient or inefficient, and they can be switched on and off. They can almost be included in the manufacturing sector.

Or so I shall argue. Before we get to that point, however, it will be necessary to discuss the difference between 'story' and 'narrative', and to introduce the idea of 'narrativity'. Later, I will consider not just jokes but illness narratives, belief in a just world, positive illusions, bad faith, and 'spirituality'. What emerges, I hope, is the idea of story-as-tool, story-as-mechanism, something with an identifiable structure which has a measurable impact on something else.

Just as the story of the camping trip has an identifiable structure – and had (I trust) a measurable impact on the reader. It made you laugh.

Definitions

The precise nature of the distinction between 'narrative' and 'story' is obscure, and there are several different accounts of it. For some writers, especially in the health care literature, the two are effectively synonymous. Where a distinction is made, it is frequently implausible. Wiltshire (1995), for example, claims that stories are 'told' while narratives are 'written'. This is puzzling because it would imply that novels and other works of fiction embody narratives but do not tell stories. Frid, et al. (2000: 695) say that 'narrative is an account of events experienced by the narrator' while storytelling is 'the repeated telling or reading of a story by persons other than narrator'. This is virtually the opposite of Wiltshire's proposal, and is baffling for a different reason: it confuses the established distinction between 'author' and 'narrator' and assumes, oddly, that all narratives are first person.

An alternative approach is more theoretical, and originates in literary criticism. According to Abbott (2002: 16), narrative 'is the representation of events, consisting of *story* and *narrative discourse*'. The idea is that a 'story' is that which is conveyed through narration. This is effectively a content/container distinction: the story is the content, while the narrative discourse – the sequence of events represented in the text or the telling – is the container. Text as ship, story as cargo. The image makes it possible to say that the same story can be told (conveyed) in different narratives (vehicles). Abbott's distinction is akin to that between *fabula* (story) and *sjuzet* (narrative ordering), introduced by Russian critics in the 1920s (Abbott, 2007), between *histoire* and *discours* (Genette, 1980), and between *story* and *discourse* (Chatman, 1978), all of which still figure in literary theory.

According to Wiltshire and Frid, then, 'narrative' and 'story' are different kinds of thing. According to literary critics, on the other hand, they are different dimensions of the same thing. However, there is a third approach, which I want to recommend here. It takes the concept of narrativity from Prince (1982), and places 'story' and 'narrative' on a continuum. Every item on this continuum counts as a narrative, but only items at one end of it count as stories. Why this is a useful way to look at the distinction will become apparent later.

Narrativity

Narrativity is something that a text has degrees of. It is possible to identify an extensive range of text features associated with narrative and place them, very roughly, in order of complexity. The simplest forms constitute 'low' narrativity; more complex forms, including stories, constitute 'high' narrativity.

Consider one definition of narrative: 'The recounting . . . of one or more real or fictitious events' (Prince, 1991: 58). It is obviously a pretty basic definition, because (as Prince concedes) it implies that a single sentence can count as an example of narrative. 'The goldfish died.' This is the recounting of one event, whether real or fictitious, so it meets the minimal requirement.

Most people, perhaps, would be inclined not to attach the label 'narrative' to this sentence, and they would be even less likely to classify it as a 'story'. However, that is not really the point. What I am proposing is that we take this initial definition as a specification of the first, and most primitive, condition that any narrative must fulfil. *No events, no narrative*. Clearly, there are more stringent conditions waiting to be identified, but this one represents the first rung on what might be called the 'ladder of narrativity' (Paley and Eva, 2005).

The number of events that must be recounted can be increased to at least two; and in fact some literary critics impose this as a formal requirement (Barthes, 1982; Rimmon-Kenan, 2002). However, this is still a very thin concept of narrative. 'The man opened the door. The goldfish died.' Two events may be an improvement on one, but we remain a long way short of what 'narrative' normally implies. Moreover, it is evident that simply piling on additional events will not help: at best, the result would just be a list of occurrences, not a narrative. What is required to take us further up the narrativity ladder is the idea of one thing leading to another, the idea that something happened because of something else.

This is the position of another group of critics (Bal, 1985; Richardson, 1997), for whom the events in a narrative must be causally related – not in a mechanistic way, but in the sense that some of them should be consequences of others. A famous literary joke illustrates the significance of this type of connection rather nicely: 'Milton wrote *Paradise Lost*, then his wife died, and then he wrote *Paradise Regained*' (Rimmon-Kenan, 2002: 17). I apologize for the sexist humour; but the point is, of course, that the joke depends on the implied causal connection between the death of Milton's wife and the title of his second epic poem.

So far, then, increasing narrativity is signified by the recounting of more than one event, some of which are causally connected. However, the Milton narrative has already added a further textual feature to this condition: it has just one central character who is critically involved in the events recounted. This is, of course, an extension of the causally-connected-events condition, which does not specify that the events in question centre on a single person. So the presence of a central character represents a further rung on the narrativity ladder (Eva and Paley, 2006).

Let me here interpolate an important observation. To say that, in a narrative, some events are causally related to others is to say that narratives make claims about causal connection. In effect, they claim (or imply) that X caused Y, that X led to Y, or that without X it is unlikely that Y would have happened. The point about such claims is that they may be true or false.

Consider the joke about Milton again. The humour, as I have suggested, depends on the implied causal connection between the death of Milton's wife and *Paradise Regained*. In effect, the claim is that her death prompted, permitted, or encouraged the writing of the poem – 'paradise' being reinterpreted as a state of happiness consequent on being no longer married. There is, of course, no reason whatsoever to suppose that this claim is true (in fact, by the time the poem was published Milton had been married to his third wife for eight years). So the causal claim, in this case, is false. Here is an alternative narrative. 'Milton was married for the first time in 1642, but his bride moved back to her parents' home not long after the wedding. Milton's first work as a married man, published in 1643, was a defence of divorce.' On this occasion, the implied causal claim is that Milton had domestic trouble, and that his experience of marriage motivated him to write *The Doctrine and Discipline of Divorce*. This time, however, there is evidence to suggest that the claim is true (Wilson, 2002).

Backtrack to the narrativity continuum. I have so far identified some preliminary conditions that must be met if a text is to count as a narrative: several events, causal connection, and a central character. But the question this has all been leading up to is: at what stage does it become legitimate to call a narrative a *story*? When does increasing narrativity take us beyond what we might call the 'story threshold'?

To some degree, the answer to this question is arbitrary. Stories may be found at the 'high narrativity' end of the continuum and not at the 'low narrativity' end; but it may be impossible to mark exactly the point at which the critical threshold is crossed. In the following section, however, I will argue that there is a textual feature which represents an especially significant upward shift in narrativity, and which – better than any other criterion – indexes the transition from bare *narrative* to full-blown *story*.

Stories

There are many instances of texts which fulfil the events-causally-connected condition which most of us would be reluctant to call stories. Examples include chronicles (as opposed to the history written by modern historians) and accounts of experiments. Even if we add a central character, as with diaries or medical case notes, calling the resulting text a story is still a bit of a stretch. However, it is possible to argue that this permutation of conditions does typify one kind of story-like narrative, namely the epic. This genre presents 'the deeds of a hero in some chronological sequence, possibly beginning with his birth, probably ending with his death' (Scholes and Kellogg, 1966: 208). As Davis (1987: 205) explains, 'Epics tend to have plots that are linked in an "and-then-and-then" fashion. This form of plot I would call "consecutive" or "causal"'. The epic, of course, belongs to the period before 1600, and since then a different kind of plot has become the norm. It is this new kind of plot that Davis terms 'teleogenic'.

The key difference between the teleogenic plot and the epic plot, or any other narrative which exhibits a purely consecutive/causal plot, is that the recounted sequence of events is, from the outset, intended to lead to a particular denouement. The narrative is given a 'shape' by the author's awareness of how it will end; and the recounted sequence of events, while still conforming to the requirements of plausible and consistent causal connection, must also be organized in such a way as to arrive at that final point. The set of circumstances with which the narrative culminates is, of course, known to the author, but not (usually) to the reader or the audience; and it is prior knowledge of this culmination which permits the author to create the narrative's structure.

Davis (1987: 206) pictures the consecutive/causal, or linear, plot in the following way:

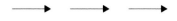

His picture of the teleogenic plot is as follows:

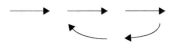

The idea of a teleogenic plot reflects the conviction, shared by numerous critics, that 'the end writes the beginning and shapes the middle' (Brooks, 1985: 22). It is what Kermode (1966) means by 'the sense of an ending', and what Sartre (1947) has in mind when he remarks that narrative proceeds 'in reverse'. In recognizing that stories have a teleogenic structure, the reader, while unaware of what the denouement will be, is nevertheless confident that there will be one, and that it will throw retrospective significance on what has preceded it. As a consequence, her making-sense-of-the-narrative activity will consist, to a considerable extent, in the 'anticipation of retrospection' (Brooks, 1985: 23).

Arguably, then, the story threshold is the point at which narrative acquires a teleogenic plot. All stories are narratives, but only teleogenic narratives are stories. As I suggested at the beginning of this chapter, jokes are where we can see this structure in its most condensed and transparent form. In a joke, the narrative is organized to culminate in the punch line, the genre's own brand of denouement. Holmes and Watson must go on a camping trip: staying in a bed and breakfast would not be helpful. The dialogue between them must take place at night, for otherwise they would presumably have been awake and noticed the theft taking place. Watson must not immediately realize that the tent has been stolen, so must be given something else to say in response to

Holmes' question – ideally something which is plausible enough to distract the audience's attention and (a bonus) set up the bathetic contrast achieved by the punch line. And so on. Narrative being constructed 'in reverse', the teleogenic plot reconciling the requirements of a plausible causal sequence with the requirements of the denouement.

Corollaries

The teleogenic plot structure has a number of consequences and corollaries, both for literary fiction and for the stories that people tell about their lives. In the remainder of this chapter, I will examine some of them, and try to indicate their significance.

Selection and editing

The requirements of a teleogenic plot are such that decisions must be made about how the story starts, what should be included and excluded, the ordering of material, and so on. If stories have 'a beginning, a middle and an end' (Gaydos, 2005; McCance, et al. 2001), this is why. In a linear narrative, such as a diary, the first and final entries represent arbitrary points in an innumerable sequence of events which comprise the diarist's life; and all the other entries reflect what the writer took to be interesting and important at the time, not a retrospective view of how some of them, with the benefit of hindsight, fit together. However, the beginning of a story is anything but arbitrary; and the events incorporated in it are selected from an indefinite range of possibilities, most of which end up being omitted because they are irrelevant to the story under construction, because they are inconsistent with it, because they fail to enhance the desired effect, or because they compromise it in some other way.

The joke about the stolen tent can again be used to illustrate these observations. The story begins as it does because (hypothetical) previous events – why Holmes and Watson decided to go camping in the first place – are irrelevant. Equally irrelevant are questions to do with the location of the camp site, why they are sharing a single tent rather than sleeping separately, how long it took Holmes to realize that the theft had taken place, and many more. Story telling of all kinds, whether fictional or autobiographical, is an extensive and ubiquitous exercise in selection and editing. This is an absolutely critical feature.

Experience

It is often suggested that experience takes a narrative form, and that we unavoidably 'grasp our lives in narrative' (Taylor, 1989: 47). This suggestion is associated with a narrative conception of the self, the idea that 'we just *are* the narrative we tell or could tell about ourselves' (Vice, 2003: 95), the view that we are characters in a story of our own making (Bruner, 1990; MacIntyre, 1982), and the claim that we lead 'storied lives' (Clandinin and Connelly, 2000). However, if the distinction between 'narrative' and 'story' adopted here is tenable, it is a mistake to run the two concepts together, as Rashotte (2005: 40), for example, does: 'To claim that we lead storied lives . . . is to assert that any experience – in order to be my experience – has narrative form'. The idea that narrative, as a recounting of causally related events, is somehow endemic to experience is not implausible; presumably, any attempt to refer to the past will involve narration in this low narrativity sense. But the theory that experience is necessarily structured by teleogenic plots, or that lives are intrinsically 'storied', is wildly overextended. Indeed, one might argue that it is barely coherent. If teleogenic plots involve *retrospective* selection, as described above, then story *cannot* be contemporary with experience; the transcendental filter through which experience is channelled. Experience is better conceived as providing the raw materials for story building. Stories, relative to experience, are very much after the fact.

At a slight tangent to the narrative conception of the self, but clearly related to it, is the often implicit idea that a narrative approach to research offers unique and authentic access to the respondent's inner world. As Atkinson (1997: 327) has pointed out, this 'sentimental and romantic version' of realism is characteristic of several writers on health and illness, especially Mishler (1984), Kleinman (1988), and Frank (1995), all of whom exhibit 'a faith in the revelatory power of the narrative' (p. 332), and expressly privilege the patient's voice at the expense of the professional's. But, as Atkinson also notes, this is to create 'a new, individualized homunculus that escapes sociological or anthropological comprehension' (p. 335), ignoring the social contexts in which narratives are forged, how they are elicited, and what their consequences are. I would merely add that teleogenic stories, the product of retrospective selection and editing, cannot possibly represent an unalloyed, authentic inner truth. They already reflect the sifting, classification, and contouring of experience. They are, in that sense, contrived.

Speech acts

More, they are contrived for a purpose. This is obvious in the case of jokes, tailored to produce a very specific outcome: laughter. But it applies to all stories: in moving towards a denouement, they create a particular emotional cadence. I will come to that idea in a moment. First, I want to briefly explore the idea that stories are a form of speech act.

As Gail Eva (Chapter 4) explains at greater length, speech act theory originates with Austin (1975), who argued that most uses of language are *performative*: they perform an action of some kind. Telling a story is what Austin calls an 'illocutionary' act, but it also has 'perlocutionary' force; that is, it has a certain effect on the audience, an effect usually intended by the author. In jokes, this is amusement. Of course, any story can be told in order to entertain; but stories can also be told with a view to moralizing, warning, convincing, scaring, impressing, attracting sympathy, instilling hope, and so on. In this sense, they are designed to manipulate those who hear them. Chambers (1984) talks of 'narrative seduction', and Phelan (2007: 209) agrees: 'narrative is a rhetorical action in which somebody tries to accomplish some purpose . . . texts are designed by authors in order to affect readers in particular ways'. In the health care context, Mattingly (1998) and Taylor (2003) adopt a similar position.

Accordingly, the most potentially useful research programme relevant to story is the determination and testing of perlocutionary effects. What impact do stories have on their audience? How is this effect achieved, and in virtue of what aspects of the story's construction? How does the audience cognitively process these structural characteristics, and with what consequences? This is the programme outlined by Bortolussi and Dixon (2003) under the slightly daunting heading *psychonarratology*. Their proposals largely concern laboratory studies; but there is enormous scope for similar research in natural settings, including health care.

Emotional cadence

The teleogenic structure of stories primes the reader for a 'promised although unpredictable outcome' (Mink,1987). 'Sherlock Holmes and Doctor Watson go on a camping trip.' Anybody hearing this will instantly recognize the schema of a joke, and will already be anticipating a punch line which somehow links an aspect of camping to the detective and his less sagacious companion. But this anticipation must be realized. If there is no punch line – if, for example, we learn only that Holmes and Watson enjoyed a splendid, sun-drenched holiday near Margate – the story will be bafflingly pointless. So the beginning of the tale provokes the expectation of a satisfying resolution to whatever story is to follow. All stories involve the creation of such expectations; good stories – ideally in unpredictable ways – fulfil them.

Velleman (2003) calls this anticipated resolution the 'emotional cadence'. Stories promise completion, just as *tick* promises *tock* (Kermode, 1966: 44). The opening line of a joke promises amusement; other stories promise different kinds of psychological consummation. Among the most familiar, one can cite: the expectation that the hero will succeed, that the boy will get the girl, that the virtuous person will be rewarded, that the villain will get his come-uppance.

These consummations are essentially normative, embodying certain kinds of preference and reflecting idealized, culturally accessible concepts of merit and desert. They represent, as Velleman (2003: 19) observes, 'patterns of how things feel', as opposed to 'patterns of how things happen'. The selection and editing required by teleogenic plots is designed, precisely, to encourage the audience to assimilate events not to the latter ('yes, that is just how things happen'), but to the *tick-tock* patterns of the former ('yes, that is just how things should feel').

This creates a potential problem. Teleogenic plots incorporate two distinct orders of explanation. The first is inherent in the causal sequence of events, and the requirement that it should be consistent and plausible (fiction), or that it should be evidenced and accurate (history and biography). The second is normative explanation, associated with the condition that exactly the same sequence of events should be resolved in an emotionally satisfying manner. This is the 'double logic' (Culler, 1981: 178) exhibited by stories, combining *cause–effect* movement with the *in-order-to-arrive-at-the-conclusion* movement. The danger, as Velleman (2003: 20) points out, is that the audience will tend to confuse the two, that it will mistake 'emotional closure for intellectual closure'. In other words, the fact that a reader finds the emotional resolution satisfying may encourage her to overlook problems in the cause – effect sequence, the narrator's claims about how one thing led to another. She may even assume that, because the story makes sense emotionally, it must also be a credible account of how things actually happened.

By way of simple illustration, let me return to the literary joke about Milton. Before I checked Milton's biography, I had imagined that when Milton wrote *Paradise Regained* he had not remarried after being widowed. My assumption was that, although the joke presumably misrepresented his feelings about his wife, what it implied about his marital situation was nevertheless accurate. It did not occur to me that this might also be a misrepresentation, despite the fact that I was writing something about the risk of confusing a satisfying resolution with a trustworthy report, which ought to have sensitized me to the possibility.

The example is a trivial but revealing one. If amusement can blind one to the question of accuracy, so can other emotions. Greater risks are attached to hearing stories which arouse sympathy or admiration. For example, in many illness narratives, the narrating patient is a 'narrative hero' and the physician is a 'narrative villain' (Atkinson, 1997: 336). Although many people who write about health care find this an emotionally satisfying typification, it would be a mistake to assume – on those grounds alone – that such narratives are necessarily credible as reports of what really occurred.

Sympathy and admiration

The emotional cadence of a teleogenic plot is almost invariably associated with the portrayal of the central character in a certain light, and the consequent elicitation of an appropriate response. This is implicit in the idea of perlocution, and is reflected in the discussion of the previous section. Stories in which the hero's virtue is rewarded invite admiration. Stories in which the central character suffers undeservedly invite sympathy. Stories which have an obvious villain invite disapproval and distaste.

First-person stories are particularly likely to exploit this function of teleogenic structure. Consider, for example, the stories we tell about ourselves. We are all familiar with the temptation to select and edit: an omission here, a little embroidery there, a subtle massaging of the facts somewhere else – with no intent to deceive, exactly, but certainly with a view to portraying ourselves as kinder, cleverer, funnier, more successful than we really are. Equally, most of us have, at one time or another, suppressed some key facts and exaggerated less important ones in order to win sympathy, playing down the extent to which failure or misfortune may have been our own responsibility, and conveying the impression that it was somebody else's (Craib, 2000). When constructed skilfully, such stories can be effective exercises in narrative seduction, the emotional cadence distracting the audience's attention away from the project of testing the causal sequence for plausibility and accuracy.

Master plots

When an author constructs a teleogenic plot, she does not usually start from scratch. As Polkinghorne (1988: 20) notes: 'Cultural traditions offer a store of plot lines which can be used to configure events into stories.' Hence the idea of a 'masterplot' (Abbott, 2002; Brooks, 1985), and the various attempts to produce a plot taxonomy (Booker, 2004; Crane, 1952; Friedman, 1975; Frye, 1957; Scholes and Kellogg, 1966). Friedman's categories, for example, include the 'admiration plot', in which an attractive hero succeeds, and so wins the reader's respect and admiration. This could also be described as the 'virtue rewarded' plot: think *Cinderella*. Another of Friedman's categories is the 'pathetic plot', in which an attractive but unfortunately weak protagonist fails, and there is an unhappy ending which provokes the reader's sympathy. These are often tales of adversity and injustice.

Many health care narratives fall into these categories. Nursing, for example, has a favourite masterplot concerning the relationship between itself and medicine. It is an example of the 'pathetic plot', in that an attractive but weak protagonist – nursing itself – succumbs to the injustices perpetrated on it by the villain (medicine), thus arousing sympathy. But one can see the shadow of the 'admiration plot' in this story, too, because nursing resembles Cinderella in her patient, put-upon virtue. Perhaps it depends on a denouement as yet unreached, with certain nurse theorists bidding for the role of fairy godmother: 'The essence of nursing is caring . . . and you *shall* go to the ball!'

Just world theory

Plot taxonomies organize stories into thematic groups: virtue rewarded, the victim, the quest, triumph against the odds, the revenge, rags to riches, and so on. At an even higher level of superordination, there are what might be termed 'meta-plots'. An example is the 'just world': a configuration of events which demonstrate that the world is ultimately a just place, and people get exactly what they deserve. The good achieve success, the bad are punished (sometimes, indirectly, by their own misdeeds). In the just world, outcomes are determined on merit.

This just world meta-plot is so deeply entrenched in western culture that, even in real life, we are very reluctant to abandon it. Indeed, during the past 40 years this reluctance has become a topic in social psychology, under the heading 'just world theory' or 'belief in a just world' (Lerner, 1980; Montada and Lerner, 1998). The theory suggests that, when confronted by circumstances which appear to disconfirm belief in a just world (BJW) – bad things happening to good people – we adopt cognitive strategies designed to preserve BJW and explain away the circumstances. One of these strategies is 'blaming the victim'. For example, in a just world, morally decent people would not contract life-limiting illnesses when young; so, if someone does contract such an illness, he cannot be morally decent (this strategy was used early in the AIDS epidemic). The contradiction is resolved by changing the appraisal of the person concerned, instead of abandoning BJW (Anderson, 1992; Braman and Lambert, 2001).

Two other strategies are more relevant to the current discussion. One is to recalibrate the bad situation, reinterpreting it as something which is in fact beneficial. In the case of illness, this implies representing suffering in a positive light, as an educative or spiritually illuminating experience (Boden and Baumeister, 1997; Mendolia, et al. 1996). The other is to embrace a belief in 'ultimate justice', supposing that, while an affliction may look unfair in the present, justice will eventually prevail, either in this world or the next (Maes, 1998; Maes and Kals, 2002). These strategies figure prominently in stories about loss. For example, people often represent the death of a partner – initially cruel and devastating – in BJW terms, through stories which claim, in effect, that it was 'a kind way to go', that they learned something from the experience, or that they will be reunited with loved ones in an afterlife (Golsworthy and Coyle, 1999).

Life as story

Earlier, I expressed scepticism about the descriptive thesis that experience takes a 'storied' form. There is also, as Vice (2003) and Strawson (2004) both observe, a normative version of the same idea. This is the view that we *should* lead 'storied lives', that 'conceiving one's life as a narrative is a good thing: a richly Narrative outlook is essential to a well-lived life' (Strawson, 2004: 428).

Vice and Strawson both take 'narrative' and 'story' as effective synonyms; and I shall not comment on the limp, and rather strange, idea that lives should be lived in *narrative* (i.e. low narrativity) mode. However, given the teleogenic view of plots adopted in this chapter, the claim that one ought, ethically, to conceptualize one's life as a *story* (high narrativity) is deeply unpersuasive. Events in the real world are part of a causal sequence; they are governed by cause and effect. They are not organized in order to arrive at conclusions; they are not 'pulled' towards denouements. So it is not evident why it should be ethically desirable to pretend that they are, which is what construing one's life as a story would mean.

If I really want to understand my life, I am confined to understanding it as events and circumstances precipitating other events and circumstances, and not as being 'drawn' towards some future state (see Lamarque, 2007 for a forceful statement of this view). In any case, the selection and editing required to invent a 'story of my life', even in retrospect, would require the exclusion of any inconvenient facts – parts of my history which did not fit the cleanly contoured, implausibly consistent teleogenic structure. It is for this reason that Craib (2000: 67) suggests: 'All personal narratives are to some degree bad faith narratives.' Iris Murdoch approaches the same idea from a slightly different angle: 'Any story which we tell about ourselves consoles us since it imposes pattern upon something which might otherwise seem intolerably chancy and incomplete. However, human life *is* chancy and incomplete.' (Murdoch, 2000: 87, emphasis added).

Positive illusions

The argument of the previous section turns on a tacit premise: that we should want to understand our lives *as they really are*, and not tell tidied-up, inevitably misleading teleogenic stories about them. But there are situations in which 'consoling ourselves', believing seductive falsehoods, may be rationally and ethically acceptable. This is a conclusion which can be drawn from the social psychological work on 'positive illusions' (Helgeson and Taylor, 1992; Taylor, et al. 2000). Studies of patients with breast cancer, heart disease, AIDS, and mental health problems have all shown that optimistic but unequivocally false beliefs are associated with enhanced health outcomes. For example, if people with HIV or diagnosed with AIDS hold unrealistically positive views about the probable trajectory of their illness, they experience less rapid disease progression and greater longevity (Reed, et al. 1994,1999) than patients whose appraisal is more realistic and accurate.

The same could be true of other forms of positive illusion – life stories, just world beliefs, spiritual and religious beliefs. In some circumstances these might be, not just examples of self-consolation, but ways of improving physical and mental health. The suggestion that religious beliefs represent a special case of 'positive illusion' has been made before (Côté and Pepler, 2005; Dennett, 2006), and it would explain the controversial research which links religion and spirituality to improved health outcomes (Koenig and Cohen, 2002; Thoresen, 1999). Here, I am more interested in 'stories about ourselves' than in religious and spiritual beliefs specifically; but in both cases it is tempting to suppose that the end of life is one situation in which the benefits of positive illusions are likely to be apparent.

Self-consolation and self-persuasion, then, turn out to be further examples of perlocutionary force. The audience for a story conceivably includes the author. So if stories are speech acts, engaged in 'narrative seduction', we can sometimes count ourselves among those we are trying to seduce (see Frank, Chapter 10).

Conclusion

Teleogenic plot structure, which I have taken to be roughly definitive of those narratives which are also stories, has remarkably fertile theoretical consequences, and the second half of this chapter has been a quick canter through its principal corollaries. The selection and editing of raw material necessitated by teleogenic plots is not carried out randomly but with a specific purpose in mind, exhibiting storytelling as a form of speech act, designed to produce a specific effect on the audience, which might include the author herself. This emotional cadence is prompted by the organization of events as a forward-looking sequence preparing for a denouement, which must be distinguished from the backward-looking causal sequence inherent in any narrative. It assimilates these events to patterns of how things should feel and, in particular, elicits familiar responses, such as sympathy and admiration, to the central character. As a result, stories can broadly be classified according to their plots, typical configurations of character and events evoking typical reactions, many of which imply the meta-plot of a 'just world'. Since stories are driven by their endings, they cannot function as a transcendental filter for experience; nor can lives be 'storied', although the pretence that they are, a form of positive illusion, can in certain circumstances be ethically justified.

At the heart of this theoretical network is the idea of narrative machinery, story-as-mechanism, a way of accomplishing a goal by telling somebody that something happened. Although jokes are the most condensed (but transient) examples of this machinery, they nevertheless reveal, in miniature, how the mechanism works. The components of the narrative, carefully selected to lead to an outcome, evoking the desired reaction. That, in a nutshell, is what stories are.

References

Abbott, H. P. (2002) *The Cambridge Introduction to Narrative*. Cambridge University Press, Cambridge, UK.

Abbott, H. P. (2007) Story, plot, and narration. In *The Cambridge Companion to Narrative* (ed. D. Herman). Cambridge University Press, Cambridge, UK, pp. 39–51.

Anderson, V. N. (1992) For whom is this world just? Sexual orientation and AIDS. *Journal of Applied Social Psychology*, **22**, 248–59.

Atkinson, P. (1997) Narrative turn or blind alley? *Qualitative Health Research*, **7**(3), 325–44.

Austin, J. L. (1975) *How To Do Things With Words*, Second Edition, Harvard University Press, Cambridge, MA.

Bal, M. (1985) *Narratology: Introduction to the Theory of Narrative*. University of Toronto Press, Toronto.

Barthes, R. (1982) Introduction to the structural analysis of narratives. In *A Barthes Reader* (ed. S. Sontag). Hill & Wang, New York, pp. 251–95.

Boden, J. M. and Baumeister, R. F. (1997) Repressive coping: Distraction using pleasant thoughts and memories. *Journal of Personality and Social Psychology*, **73**, 45–62.

Booker, C. (2004) *The Seven Basic Plots: Why We Tell Stories*. Continuum, London.

Bortolussi, M. and Dixon, P. (2003) *Psychonarratology: Foundations for the Empirical Study of Literary Response*. Cambridge University Press, Cambridge, UK.

Braman, A. C. and Lambert, A. J. (2001) Punishing individuals for their infirmities. Effects of personal responsibility, just-world beliefs, and in-group/out-group status. *Journal of Applied Social Psychology*, **31**, 1096–109.

Brooks, P. (1985) *Reading for Plot*. Random House, New York.

Bruner, J. (1990) *Acts of Meaning*. Harvard University Press, Cambridge, MA.

Chambers, R. (1984) *Story and Situation: Narrative Seduction and the Power of Fiction*. Manchester University Press, Manchester, UK.

Chatman, S. (1978) *Story and Discourse: Narrative Structure in Fiction and Film*. Cornell University Press, Ithaca.

Clandinin, D. J. and Connelly, F. M. (2000) *Narrative Inquiry: Experience and Story in Qualitative Research*. Jossey-Bass, San Francisco.

Côté, J. K. and Pepler, C. (2005) A focus for nursing intervention: Realistic acceptance or helping illusions? *International Journal of Nursing Practice*, **11**, 39–43.

Craib, I. (2000) Narrative as bad faith. In *Lines of Narrative: Psychosocial Perspectives* (eds. M. Andrews, S. D. Sclater, C. Squire and A. Treacher). Routledge, London, pp. 64–74.

Crane, R. S. (1952) The concept of plot and the plot of Tom Jones. In *Critics and Criticism*, Abridged Edition, (ed. R. S. Crane). University of Chicago Press, Chicago, pp. 62–93.

Culler, J. (1981) *The Pursuit of Signs*. Routledge and Kegan Paul, London.

Davis, L. J. (1987) *Resisting Novels: Ideology and Fiction*. Methuen, London.

Dennett, D. (2006) *Breaking the Spell*. Penguin, London.

Eva, G. and Paley, J. (2006) Stories in palliative care. *Progress in Palliative Care*, **14**(4), 155–64.

Frank, A. W. (1995) *The Wounded Storyteller: Body, Illness and Ethics*. University of Chicago Press, Chicago.

Frid, I., Öhlén, J. and Bergbom, I. (2000) On the use of narratives in nursing research. *Journal of Advanced Nursing*, **32**(3), 695–703.

Friedman, N. (1975) *Form and Meaning in Fiction*. University of Georgia Press, Athens.

Frye, N. (1957) *The Anatomy of Criticism*. Princeton University Press, Princeton, NJ.

Gaydos, H. L. (2005) Understanding personal narratives: An approach to practice. *Journal of Advanced Nursing*, **49**(3), 254–59.

Genette, G. (1980) *Narrative Discourse: An Essay on Method*. Cornell University Press, Ithaca.

Golsworthy, R. and Coyle, A. (1999) Spiritual beliefs and the search for meaning among older adults following partner loss. *Mortality*, **4**(1), 21–40.

Helgeson, V. S. and Taylor, S. E. (1992) Social comparisons and adjustment among cardiac patients. *Journal of Applied Social Psychology*, **23**, 1171–95.

Kermode, F. (1966) *The Sense of an Ending: Studies in the Theory of Fiction*. Oxford University Press, Oxford.

Kleinman, A. (1988) *The Illness Narratives: Suffering, Healing and the Human Condition*. Basic Books, New York.

Koenig, H. G. and Cohen, H. J. (eds) (2002) *The Link Between Religion and Health: Psychoneuroimmunology and the Faith Factor*. Oxford University Press, Oxford.

Lamarque, P. (2007) On the distance between literary narratives and real-life narratives. In *Narrative and Understanding Persons* (ed. D. D. Hutto). Cambridge University Press, Cambridge, UK, pp. 117–32.

Lerner, M. J. (1980) *The Belief in a Just World: A Fundamental Delusion*. Plenum Press, New York.

MacIntyre, A. (1982) *After Virtue*. Duckworth, London.

Maes, J. (1998) Immanent justice and ultimate justice: Two ways of believing in justice. In *Responses to Victimizations and Belief in a Just World* (eds. L. Montada, and M. J. Lerner). Plenum, New York, pp. 9–40.

Maes, J. and Kals, E. (2002) Justice beliefs in school: Distinguishing ultimate and immanent justice. *Social Justice Research*, **15**, 227–44.

Mattingly, C. (1998) *Healing Dramas and Clinical Plots: The Narrative Structure of Experience*. Cambridge University Press, Cambridge.

McCance, T. V., McKenna, H. P., and Boore, J. R. P. (2001) Exploring caring using narrative methodology: An analysis of the approach. *Journal of Advanced Nursing*, **33**(3), 350–56.

Mendolia, M., Moore, J., and Tesser, A. (1996) Dispositional and situational determinants of repression. *Journal of Personality and Social Psychology*, **70**, 856–67.

Mink, L. O. (1987) History and fiction as modes of comprehension. In *Historical Understanding* (eds. B. Fay, E. O. Golob, and R. T. Vann). Cornell University Press, Ithaca.

Mishler, E. G. (1984) *The Discourse of Medicine*. Ablex, Norwood, NJ.

Montada, L. and Lerner, M. J. (eds) (1998) *Responses to Victimizations and belief in a Just World*. Plenum, New York.

Murdoch, I. (2000) *The Sovereignty of the Good*. Routledge, London.

Paley, J. and Eva, G. (2005) Narrative vigilance: The analysis of stories in health care. *Nursing Philosophy*, **6**(2), 83–97.

Phelan, J. (2007) Rhetoric/ethics. In *The Cambridge Companion to Narrative* (ed. D. Herman). Cambridge University Press, Cambridge, UK, pp. 203–16.

Polkinghorne, D. (1988) *Narrative Knowing and the Human Sciences*. State University of New York Press, Albany.

Prince, G. (1982) *Narratology: The Form and Functioning of Narrative*. Mouton, Berlin.

Prince, G. (1991) *Dictionary of Narratology*. Scolar Press, Aldershot.

Rashotte, J. (2005) Dwelling with stories that haunt us: Building a meaningful nursing practice. *Nursing Inquiry*, **12**(1), 34–42.

Reed, G. M., Kemeny, M. E., Taylor, S. E., and Visscher, B. R. (1999) Negative HIV-specific explanations and AIDS-related bereavement as predictors of symptom onset in asymptomatic HIV-positive gay men. *Health Psychology*, **18**, 354–63.

Reed, G. M., Kemeny, M. E., Taylor, S. E., Wang, H.-Y. J., and Visscher, B. R. (1994) 'Realistic acceptance' as a predictor of decreased survival time in gay men with AIDS. *Health Psychology*, **13**, 299–307.

Richardson, B. (1997) *Unlikely Stories: Causality and the Nature of Modern Narrative*. University of Delaware Press, Newark, DE.

Rimmon-Kenan, S. (2002) *Narrative Fiction*. Second Edition, Routledge, London.

Sartre, J.-P. (1947) *La Nausée*. Gallimard, Paris.

Scholes, R. and Kellogg, R. (1966) *The Nature of Narrative*. Oxford University Press, London.

Strawson, G. (2004) Against narrativity. *Ratio*, **17**(4), 428–52.

Taylor, C. (1989) *The Sources of the Self*. Cambridge University Press, Cambridge, UK.

Taylor, C. (2003) Narrating practice: Reflective accounts and the textual construction of reality. *Journal of Advanced Nursing*, **42**(3), 244–51.

Taylor, S. E., Kemeny, M. E., Reed, G. M., Bower, J. E., and Gruenewald, T. L. (2000) Psychological resources, positive illusions, and health. *American Psychologist*, **55**(1), 99–109.

Thoresen, C. E. (1999) Spirituality and health: Is there a relationship? *Journal of Health Psychology*, **4**, 291–300.

Velleman, J. D. (2003) Narrative explanation. *The Philosophical Review*, **112**(1), 1–25.

Vice, S. (2003) Literature and the narrative self. *Philosophy*, **78**, 93–108.

Wilson, A. N. (2002) *A Life of John Milton*. Pimlico, London.

Wiltshire, J. (1995) Telling a story, writing a narrative: Terminology in health care. *Nursing Inquiry*, **2**, 75–82.

Chapter 2

The possibilities of narrative palliative care medicine: 'Giving Sorrow Words'

Sayantani DasGupta, Craig Irvine, and Maura Spiegel

Give sorrow words. The grief that does not speak
Whispers the o'er fraught heart and bids it break.
Shakespeare, *Macbeth*, Act IV Scene 3

We die. That may be the meaning of life. But we *do*
language. That may be the measure of our lives.
Toni Morrison, *Morrison, 1993*

'Gentleman,' he said, 'Ivan Ilych has died!' 'You don't say so!' 'Here, read it yourself,' replied Peter Ivanovich, handing Fëdor Vasilievich the paper still damp from the press (Tolstoy 2006). Our scene opens in a hospital. Not Tolstoy's Russia, but a modern day temple of healing. Perhaps we are with medical students in the conference room whose walls are lined with somber portraits of white-coated physicians. Perhaps we are with residents on an inpatient floor, in a room scattered with leftover doughnuts, half-written progress notes, an X-Ray still mounted on the view box. Perhaps we are in a room of doctors, nurses, chaplains, and hospital staff members, who have come together during their noon lunch hour to study literature.

We are in a place of life and death, and we are *doing* language. We are reading together *The Death of Ivan Ilych*, Tolstoy's classic short novel about the meaning of an authentic life and a good death. When we read this novel in the Program in Narrative Medicine at Columbia University—during a student humanities course, during residents' narrative rounds, or during our monthly literature at work sessions—we often begin by discussing why Tolstoy would announce Ivan's death at the beginning of his novel. Most novels do not reveal the ultimate fate of their central characters until late in their stories, building suspense around such central issues as who will live and who will die. Indeed, delayed revelation is more typical of Tolstoy himself: we don't learn of Anna Karenina's doom, for example, until very late in the novel, Tolstoy narrating us to her death "as it happens," so to speak. So why, we ask our readers, is Tolstoy so revealing in the title, removing all suspense about whether or not his central character will die? Inevitably, among the first answers we receive is some version of the following: "It seems as if Tolstoy tells us right away so that we're not distracted by our curiosity. That way he forces us to focus on the process of dying itself." This perspective—this focus on the process of dying—is one that clinicians are not used to adopting. Death, we believe, lies *outside* medicine's story. As soon as it becomes apparent that death is inevitable, medicine has no further role to play and so must take its leave.

It is precisely for this reason that we at the Program in Narrative Medicine read *The Death of Ivan Ilych* in our work with clinicians; it is precisely for this reason that we read and write with clinicians. Central to our work is that we *do* language together—examining together papers "still damp from the press," opening ourselves up to each other's readings of literature, to each other's intimate writings, and to each other's interpretations of life and death—for the purposes of living our lives as clinicians and caring for our patients more fully.

The Program in Narrative Medicine at Columbia University is based on the premise that the care of the sick unfolds in stories; that individuals experiencing illness need to share their narratives, and clinicians need to listen fully. Caregivers have stories too, and voicing these stories helps them more fully understand, experience, and deliver care to those who are sick. The Program in Narrative Medicine trains health care professionals and trainees in many disciplines: medicine, nursing, social work, physical therapy, occupational therapy, psychoanalysis, pastoral care. In addition, it offers workshops and services for patients and families experiencing illness.

Explicitly interdisciplinary, our program has drawn together individuals who are themselves working at the interstices of multiple disciplines. The authors of this chapter are three of the core faculty of the Program in Narrative Medicine; we are a philosopher and family medicine educator (CI), a literature and film scholar (MS), and a pediatrician and memoirist (SD). Although our clinical education and training endeavors inevitably address some aspects of death and dying, none of the authors is explicitly involved in either palliative care education or training. Therefore, we approach this collaboratively written essay with a collaborative agenda. While we are interested in sharing our own insights in narrative medicine that may be useful in both palliative care practice and education, we are also interested in looking to palliative care as a model for narrative practice in medicine.

Death and the plot of medicine

Narrative is not, of course, new to medicine. For centuries, stories have been considered the building blocks of relationships between clinicians and patients, who were also often members of the same community. Outside of quite rural settings, however, such a model of medical practice is rarely the norm today. Urbanization has occurred side by side with the mechanization of medicine. Modern day physicians are therefore rarely tied to their patients by shared community stories. Simultaneously, medical practice has shifted away from a focus on individual narratives and relationships to situations where patients might see a series of providers who are equipped with the most modern technologies of diagnosis and treatment. With great strides in curing disease have come great dangers to the profession: the potential for impersonal care, unsatisfactory relationships, and ultimately, a disappointment in medicine on the part of both its practitioners and its patients (Frank, 2004a).

These historical changes in a narrative-based medicine parallel broader cultural as well as professional changes in attitude towards mourning and death. Physicians rarely mourn with the families of their deceased patients, occasionally even neglecting to acknowledge the death itself. Consider, for instance, that in nineteenth-century America, the doctor's letter of condolence was an important part of the support offered to the family of the deceased patient. In the following 1892 letter, as quoted in *The New England Journal of Medicine* in 2001, the physician's role as friend and fellow mourner is made obvious. The letter also testifies to the critical importance of story—the story told in the letter itself about the patient, as well as Dr Jackson's reference to the patient's stor(i)es of "wit and wisdom":

> My Dear Friend,
> I need not tell you how much I have sympathized with you. I think I realize in some measure how much you will miss dear Aunt Nancy for a long time—for the rest of your life. I know that she has been a part of you. . . . Mind as well as body was duly exercised, and she always had stock from which she poured out stores for the delight of her friends,—stores of wit and wisdom, affording pleasure with profit to all around her.
>
> How constantly will the events of life recall her to our minds—realizing what she said or did under interesting and important circumstance—or perhaps suggesting imperfectly what she would have said under new and unexpected occurrences.

For you my dear friend I implore God's blessing.
Your old friend,

J. Jackson (Bedell, et al. 2001)

Western medical attitudes to death are shaped by broader cultural contexts. With the shift of death at the beginning of the twentieth century from the home and community to the hospital, death itself became professionalized and lost its place in the plot of life. In the words of the historian Philippe Aries (1974: 69), "Death . . . ceased to be accepted as a natural, necessary phenomenon. Death is a failure, a 'business lost'. . . . When death arrives, it is regarded as an accident, a sign of helplessness or clumsiness that must be put out of mind" (quoted in Laderman, 2003: 4). Similarly, in his now classic *The Wounded Storyteller,* sociologist Arthur Frank has suggested that, in the late twentieth and early twenty-first century, the pervasive Western illness narrative is the "restitution narrative." In Frank's words, "contemporary culture treats health as the normal condition that people ought to have restored." The plot of restitution is characterized by the expectation that "yesterday I was healthy, today I'm sick, but tomorrow I'll be healthy again" (Frank, 1995: 77). This is a narrative that is institutionally, as well as individually, perpetuated. Indeed, the restitution narrative in many ways supports the power of medicine itself, since the expectation on the part of both patients and practitioners is that, through the surrendering of the ill individual to the institution of medicine, that person may be restored to the pre-illness self.

Consider the following story recently told by a resident to one of the authors (CI) at Columbia University Center for Family and Community Medicine's inpatient Narrative Medicine rounds. The author asked the residents, medical students, and attending physicians on the service that day to write about the experiences that most shaped the way they view death. We then took turns reading aloud what we had written. One of the residents, Monica, was visibly distressed when it was her turn to share. As a devout Christian, Monica told the group, she was absolutely convinced—has indeed never doubted—that death was a doorway to a better, more glorious existence. In accordance with Monica's faith, death was to be accepted, even welcomed, as God's divine will. As a doctor, however, Monica experienced every death as something shameful, something wrong. She got angry every time one of her patients died, berating herself with a question all too familiar to every doctor in the room that day: "Why did this have to happen on my watch?!" Monica could not seem to help feeling that every death was a failure, in spite of the fact that this is so clearly at odds with the most deeply cherished values of her spiritual tradition. This conflict between her spiritual and professional values was very painful for Monica. She could not see a way to reconcile her belief that death is part of life—even part of the divine order—with the message inculcated by her medical training: death is always the enemy, to be battled with every weapon in one's medical arsenal.

Clearly, despite Susan Sontag's (Sontag, 1988) cautions to the contrary, military metaphors continue to shape clinical practice. The construction of physician as soldier, hospital as front line, and death as the enemy is still extraordinarily common in medical education and training. Until recently, few medical schools or residency training programs included any palliative care education, and attitudes toward terminally ill and dying patients are still most often learned through the hidden curriculum—as modeled by senior medical staff. Consider the educational messages of the story shared above: "Not on my watch" is an oft-heard mantra of house staff in an environment where death during one's shift is considered a failure.

These limitations placed on stories are not solely individual choices: they are built into the very systems of medicine. Consider the struggle described by general internist and writer Rafael Campo, whose desire to connect with his patient's death beyond "the facts" is thwarted by structural expectations that he, as a physician, stay within literal and metaphoric lines of what has become considered the standard of physician professionalism:

> A patient of mine died recently, and as I dutifully filled out his death certificate beneath a sputtering fluorescent light in my hospital's admitting office, I wondered about the tales we tell in medicine and what purposes they serve. In the block print and black ink required by the form, I wrote "RESPIRATORY ARREST" and then "CHRONIC OBSTRUCTIVE PULMONARY DISEASE." As I signed it, I felt how woefully inadequate was the summary I had just provided. Yet there were no blanks on the standard legal document for explaining the patient's chronic pain or for describing his faded tattoos or recounting his penchant for New York-style cheesecake—and surely for good reason: the Commonwealth of Massachusetts was interested in him purely for statistical and demographic purposes. I slipped the form unceremoniously into the appropriate folder and headed for the exit. Whether I should attend his funeral and what to say to his longtime partner, also my patient, at his next visit were my problems. . . . I say "problems" because we in the medical profession seldom, if ever, give much thought to what lies beyond the clearly drawn boundaries of our clinical engagement with our patients.
>
> (Campo, 2004: 1014)

Current attempts to reintroduce condolence letters to an increasingly impersonal medical practice (Bedell, et al. 2001) or acknowledge the importance of the physician's presence at funerals (Irvine, 1985) can be understood as narrative struggles. In other words, they are attempts to reinsert the physician into the life narrative of the patient—a narrative that, when defined broadly, extends beyond the biological life of the patient to include his death, and the impact of that death upon his loved ones and community. The diagnostic dilemma, then, lies in the realm of the story. If the stories that we, as a broader culture and a particular professional discipline, tell about our lives are predominantly restitution narratives, then there is little room in such tales for death. The challenge, then, is no less than to critically examine and understand the stories we tell, as a culture, as a profession, about life, and to reinsert death within that story, not solely as an ending, but as Tolstoy suggested, as part of the ongoing story's plot. Here is where palliative care can be used as a model for the rest of narrative medical practice.

While this rather Herculean task is being accomplished, what can narrative medicine offer palliative care? In other words, why should practitioners caring for terminally ill and dying patients practice *narrative palliative care medicine*?

Narrative palliative care medicine

In our work in the Program in Narrative Medicine, we have been involved in the development of many programs in various clinical disciplines. Indeed, there is no longer one singular discipline called "Narrative Medicine" but rather a series of interconnected disciplines: narrative internal medicine, narrative pediatrics, narrative genetics, narrative geriatrics, and so on. In that vein, what does a narratively based palliative care look like? What qualities distinguish it from a *non-narratively based* practice of palliative care?

Historically, the notion of the 'good death' has been central to the palliative and hospice care movements. This idea is inherently narrative in its nature and not unrelated in fact to Tolstoy's notion in *The Death of Ivan Ilych* that the "good death" might arise from a spiritually fulfilled "authentic" life. Most often, the modern "good death" is related to the expectation that dying individuals are given an opportunity to recall and share/review their life stories, resolving "unfinished business" and accepting impending death (Baugher, 2008).

Yet narrative medicine, including narrative palliative care medicine, must be committed to a constant self-critique regarding such issues as the authorship of stories, expectations regarding stories, and responsibility to stories. Indeed, many who are writing and thinking in the arena of hospice care have critiqued the notion of the "good death" and the "good death story." The term itself gives rise to multiple lines of inquiry: by whose definition are we to judge a "good death"? How does an individual's particular subject position—her gender, sexuality, ethnicity, culture, religion, nationality—influence her ability to have a "good death?" How are we to understand the semi-examined or unexamined death—the "good enough death" or even the "bad death?"

Sociologist John Baugher (2008) has described the tension between the dying person's authority over the story—and indeed her right to tell or not tell—and the palliative care worker's responsibility as an 'expert' to facilitate the "good death story." Indeed, Baugher points to the conflation of the term "listening" with "facilitating" among hospice workers. He suggests that "grief work" has become operationalized to the point that dying people have been "constructed as a type of worker with 'tasks' to complete," and that, in this context, "the need for a professional class to facilitate those tasks seems natural" (Baugher, 2008: 3). Here, we see palliative care encountering the same narrative challenges as other disciplines: faced with the requirement of listening to stories, listening itself becomes operationalized to the point of meaninglessness. Thinking we are being 'professional,' we nod, smile, and give encouraging noises indicating we are listening, in a hollow imitation of the original act we intended to undertake.

Another stumbling block encountered by many clinical disciplines is the expectation that the narrative itself is an object—a "thing" that exists within defined boundaries—rather than understanding narratives as intrinsically relational events that are born between a particular teller and a particular listener at a particular point in time. As Arthur Frank (2004b) asserts, illness stories are necessarily social; even stories without a flesh and blood listener imply a potential witness, whose identity, be it doctor, family member, or fellow sufferer, helps shape the form and content of the story itself.

Indeed, the expectation that this final, unalterable "thing" narrative can or should be somehow obtained suggests the expectation that in understanding this definitive story, the dying individual can also be understood (see also Gunaratnam, Chapter 3). In other words, the story becomes an approximation for the patient. This expectation is vexed. The philosopher Emmanuel Levinas suggested that the Other lies always and necessarily beyond the comprehension of the Self. Endeavors to fully capture, understand or master the Other are, therefore, no more than totalizing enterprises—attempts to impose my self on the Other, to bring the Other into my domain. For Levinas, the primordial ethical act lies in answering the call of the suffering Other; answering the call of the Other whom we can never fully know but to whom we are ultimately responsible (Irvine, 2005). In expecting that we can somehow capture the patient's 'true' narrative and 'true' self, we risk our clinical practice becoming one of mastery.

In his text *The Illness Narratives,* Arthur Kleinman (1988) describes the story of Gordon Stuart, a 33-year-old writer dying of metastasized rectal cancer, and his doctor, Hadley Eliot, a hospice physician who has been visiting Stuart at home, providing palliation for his pain, and witness for his story. Kleinman transcribes a taped recording of one of their visits, which occurred ten days before Gordon Stuart died. Although Gordon Stuart is a writer, and aware of the power of written narrative, he describes being too exhausted to write by the "me/not me" that is his body's cancer. What happens instead is that his oral narrative emerges specifically and necessarily from his relationship with his physician. This narrative allows him to organize his experience, grant meaning to his life's events, and approach death "midsentence . . . with the best part left unsaid." Kleinman quotes the exchange as follows:

> Gordon: . . . I've been trying to write down my feelings. But I simply don't have the energy or the concentration. . . . I forget what I've gone through. The inexorable course of things. The feeling there is something not me in me, an "it," eating its way through the body. I am the creator of my own destruction. These cancer cells are me and yet not me. I am invaded by a killer. I am become death. I really don't want to die. I know I must. I will. I am. But I don't want to.
>
> (There is another long silence.)
>
> Hadley: Do you want me to turn this tape recorder off?
>
> Gordon: No, don't. This helps me feel I will leave something behind. Not quite up to the vaulting ambition I've had, but something nonetheless. . . . I want to thank you, Hadley, for the time you have spent, the things you have done. I know I couldn't be here without you. I couldn't take dying in a hospital. It goes against the grain of everything I value: nature, home, life, that which is human and tender. Thank you, Hadley.
>
> Hadley: It's you who is doing it, Gordon.
>
> Gordon: I know that. No one can die for me. . . . I want to talk about something else, Hadley.
>
> Hadley: Go ahead, Gordon, I've got time. I'd like to hear.
>
> Gordon: I think too much can be made of death. . . . But some moments like this, I feel ready to make an end, a final stop. We come into life, we spend an awful long time growing up, and then we go.. . . . Death perhaps is the meaning of life. Only when we think of it in the real terms of our death do we realize this is the ultimate relevance. You see, Hadley, death is making me into a philosopher. Maybe it's because you are such a good listener and I get such a good feeling after talking to you. I think I'm ready, Hadley. If I could will it, I would die now—in midsentence, ironically, with the best part left unsaid. You can go now, Hadley. You've done good today.
>
> (Kleinman, 1988: 148–9)

Kleinman suggests that the most remarkable quality of the interview is the "participants' struggle to maintain authenticity, to avoid sentimentalizing or in other ways rendering inauthentic a relationship centered on the most existential of problems" (Kleinman, 1988: 153). Kleinman points out that the physician has no answers for the dying patient, nor does the dying patient seek them. Rather, what the physician provides here is what Kleinman calls "empathetic witnessing," asserting that this witnessing is "not a technical procedure" (Kleinman, 1988: 154). Indeed, this exchange is the achievement of both parties who have nurtured a mutual trust over the course of time, and clearly it provided comfort not only to Gordon Stuart, the dying man, but to Hadley Eliott, the physician. If the depth of their connection intensified the loss experienced by the caregiver, it also affirmed the meaning of his work, in its deepest value. Ultimately, if we understand clinical stories, in any discipline, as not "things," but as relational events—as profound experiences rather than professional "work"—we begin to approach a narratively based practice.

Attention, representation, affiliation

Rita Charon, founder and director of the Program in Narrative Medicine, coined the term "narrative competence" in order to make explicit the need for clinicians to have narrative skills or, in the parlance of educational milestones, competencies. The central triumvirate of such narrative competence, she has written, may be termed attention, representation, and affiliation (Charon, 2006).

Attention refers to the witnessing function which is so critical to any clinical relationship. In such witnessing, the clinician is deeply and entirely present to and for the patient's story. This suggests a profoundly different sort of practice than that of someone who has been taught a checklist of listening indicators—nodding, smiling, and the like (see Stanworth, this volume). In the words of John Berger, author of *A Fortunate Man: The Story of a Country Doctor* (1997), the central work of the physician is that of recognition:

> This individual and closely intimate recognition is required on both a physical and psychological level. On the former it constitutes the art of diagnosis. Good general diagnosticians are rare, not because most doctors lack medical knowledge, but because most are incapable of taking in all the possibly relevant facts—emotional, historical, environmental as well as physical. They are searching for specific conditions instead of the truth about a man which may then suggest various conditions. (p. 73)

The receptivity of attention can place the practitioner in a position of being 'acted upon', seemingly antithetical to the activity that defines professional practice in medicine. Consider the following point, made by one of the authors in another essay:

> If anything, medicine acts—it examines, interprets, investigates, scans, incises, de-briefs and sutures. In grammatical terms, almost all of medical practice occurs in the active voice. By this I refer to the voice of a verb which "denotes whether the subject performs or receives the action expressed by the verb." The active voice "shows the subject as actor" as opposed to the passive voice which "shows the subject as acted upon" (Phillips June 17, 1985). Here, then, is one small beacon illuminating the crisis of story in medicine. If subjecthood in the medical profession is predicated on assuming an active voice in most professional activities—doing things—then it only follows that medical subjects—namely, physicians—should approach the witnessing of stories from a similar stance. We speak of "getting the story" as if it were an object

to be found and fetched intact, an active, even athletic, process of discovery, archaeology, search-and-rescue. Yet, the witnessing of suffering is nothing if not a process of being "acted upon," humbled, changed and filled in addition to being informed. And so, this sort of listening demands a radical shift in stance—in grammatical "voice"—such that physicians not only act but allow themselves to be acted upon.

(DasGupta, 2007: 1385)

Indeed, Dame Cicely Saunders, the founder of the modern hospice movement, drew from the origins of the word "hospice" (*hospes*)—in Latin both "host" and "guest"—to suggest the importance of mutuality in the palliative care relationship (Baugher, 2008). In other words, even as the witness is being with another in his suffering, she is simultaneously being given the gift of the sufferer being with her. Rather than a professional facilitator who is tasked with assisting in "grief work," the witness becomes an equal player in the mutual experience of storytelling and storylistening, but she is also a witness with responsibilities. "What is this I have witnessed?" the physician must ask herself, "and what does it mean?" Such self-reflection demands that the physician be aware and alert to her own cadre of personal and professional stories that may influence her to hear and be present for one sort of narrative and dismiss or distort another. This sort of self-awareness is particularly critical in palliative care work, where deep-seeded anxieties, hopes, fears, and sorrows are undoubtedly brought up in the practitioner – listener relationship.

In a forthcoming article, one of the authors (CI) relays a story written by a fourth-year medical student, Ashley, for his elective narrative ethics course. The story is about a patient named Mary, who was not much older than Ashley. On the first morning of Ashley's first inpatient rotation, Mary was hospitalized with sepsis, caused by immune suppression from chemotherapy. Ashley's story is particularly revelatory of the way that medical training shapes the attitudes toward death of medical professionals:

> Shortly after arriving on the floor, Mary developed Acute Respiratory Distress Syndrome. . . . [T]he Chief Resident told Ashley to sit by the bed and encourage Mary to relax. For more than five hours, while residents and attendings ran in and out of the room doing everything in their power to arrest Mary's respiratory decline, Ashley held Mary's hand, repeating, over and over again, "Just breathe. Relax, it's going to be okay. . . ." When Mary stopped breathing, the Chief Resident pushed Ashley away from the bed, and he and the rest of the team began the code. Death was declared several minutes later. The team abruptly left the room, leaving Ashley alone with Mary's battered body. No one ever spoke to her about Mary's death.

> When Ashley finished reading this story to me, she looked up and said, through her tears and without irony, "I just wish I'd been able to do something for Mary, like everyone else. I felt so helpless. Just useless and in the way." In the two years since Mary's death, Ashley had never shared this story with anyone at her school.

The author then relays the ways that writing, reading and discussing her story helped to orient Ashley to a new perspective on a deeply painful event:

> During our discussion, we considered the role the "character" of the medical student plays in the story of Mary's death. In this story, Ashley discovered, the student plays a much more important role than any of the doctors: Mary would have died whether or not Ashley was there, but her death would have been far less peaceful. While the importance of Ashley's role seemed immediately obvious to me, as it would to most readers of her story, Ashley had not, previously, been encouraged to acknowledge the moral authority of her actions. On the contrary, her professional training had actively discouraged this acknowledgement. . . . Writing and sharing her story offered Ashley a means of memorializing Mary's death—a means of preserving the memory, and so placing the meaning, of an event radically dislocated by her professional training.
>
> (Irvine, 2009)

In this process of representation—writing about a patient, sharing the written text and allowing for responses and discussion—a number of purposes are served that, we propose, assist caregivers in contending with the tasks they routinely perform. Only in *writing about* this experience and through the discussion that followed, did Ashley discover the value in her actions on that day two years earlier. In putting words down on paper, in conferring form upon a previously unspoken experience, she located a relation to it; she "placed the meaning." In our work in Narrative Medicine, we find that writing, constructing a poem or short narrative, gives shape and context to experience, providing the writer access to experiences which—without a self-imposed form—could prove potentially overwhelming. Entering into a feeling by employing creative resources or simply different sources of knowledge than those deployed in the medical setting helps caregivers build strategies for addressing difficult emotions and for responding to others. A piece of writing, even one written in just a few short minutes, can perform a weighty and worthy function as memorial, as a site of remembrance.

Finding a "place" for death in both the physician's and patient's life stories requires and creates narrative community. Julia E. Connelly writes that "One shared story triggers the telling of other stories by involved listeners, facilitates memories and personal reflections on past experiences,. . . and creates an expanded awareness. . . of personal presence and connectedness" (Connelly, 2002: 145). This "expanded awareness" is in evidence whenever medical practitioners gather to share their stories. In every story shared, the community of storytellers discovers and creates connections—affiliations— to all of the other stories, thus building upon and reinforcing a communal narrative coherence.

Indeed, in our current work in the Program in Narrative Medicine, we have found the demand for narrative training and narrative outlet emerging organically from students, patient groups, health care organizations, and clinical teams. For example, a few years ago, our program was approached by Gwen Nichols, the then director of the Hematological Malignancy Program at Columbia, with a serious problem. There had been a devastating death on the adult oncology inpatient unit: a pregnant woman with a brain tumor whose foetus had died as well. The oncology team—nurses, doctors, administrators—was beyond disheartened. Indeed, the death actually prompted one of the residents to consider leaving the profession of medicine entirely, saying "I can't do this." In response to this crisis, a twice monthly lunchtime elective writing seminar was created—the "narrative oncology" project—as an effort to both decrease burn-out and increase understanding and affiliation among clinical team members. The interdisciplinary group has been in existence now for over five years, sharing difficult and intimate writing, inviting collective insight into personal experience, and building team collegiality and commitment. Importantly, the traditional hospital hierarchy, whereby information and insight flows only "downhill"—from more powerful to less powerful players—becomes overturned, such that a senior oncology attending physician may have his writing witnessed and given interpretive insight by a junior level nurse in training. Since writing often emerges from care of common patients, the group allows for a multivocal medicine whereby the group can take multiple points of view on one situation, an experience that challenges the dominance of any one perspective over another (Charon, 2006).

Conclusion

A recent essay in the *New England Journal of Medicine* on teaching palliative medicine at Harvard begins with the following observation from by a student:

> I thought I would find out what death actually is. I thought I would learn the proper words to speak. . . . I thought I would leave with answers to my questions about the end of life and how people cope with dying. . . . I hoped there would be a protocol to follow when a patient dies that would protect me from the suffering and grief. My experiences throughout this course have proven to me that to have answers to these questions would make me nonhuman.
>
> (Mauro Zappaterra, Harvard Medical School, Class of 2007 [Block and Billings, 2005: 1313])

A similar sentiment was expressed not long ago at our biannual weekend workshop in Narrative Medicine when a clinician shared a memory that she said has haunted her for 30 years. She wrote about a day when, as a third-year medical student, she was told to remain with a patient, a youngish woman, who was still unconscious following oncological surgery. The operation had quite literally been "open and shut" as the surgeon had found the woman's tumor and metastases too wide-spread for operative treatment.

The clinician stood by, and in a few moments the woman began to stir. Opening her eyes, the patient looked at the author and asked, "Am I dying?" The written account did not include the answer the physician gave. What was implicit was her sense of failure in that moment, as she simply had no idea what to say. Even to this day, now a well-established teacher, the physician is still struggling with this story. Is there, after all, any kind of technical or skill-training, any pre-packaged language to prepare one for such a moment? The contention of Narrative Medicine is that in developing and deepening strategies for attending, representing and affiliating with patients and with colleagues, caregivers gain confidence in their ability to face their own fears and dread of just such an inassimilable moment. It is the aspiration of Narrative Medicine to help caregivers develop the confidence that they will find an answer for a patient like the one described above—that is, that they will cultivate the combination of *humility* (DasGupta, 2008) and confidence called for in such a moment—to be present in oneself.

At the end of *The Death of Ivan Ilych*, the protagonist embraces his own mortality and accepts the inevitability of his death. In doing so, the fear of death he once knew is undone and something else is put in its place. Narrative palliative care medicine has the potential to alter the rest of medicine's relationship with death, whereby death is placed once more in life's ongoing plot, whereby physicians no longer fear death but see the joy in living with the stories of their patients, and the stories of themselves. Writes Tolstoy:

"And death. . . where is it?"

He sought his former accustomed fear of death and did not find it. "Where is it? What death?" There was no fear because there was no death.

In place of death there was light.

"So that's what it is!" he suddenly exclaimed aloud. "What joy!"

To him all this happened in a single instant, and the meaning of that instant did not change. For those present his agony continued for another two hours. Something rattled in his throat, his emaciated body twitched, then the gasping and rattle became less and less frequent.

"It is finished!" said someone near him.

He heard these words and repeated them in his soul.

"Death is finished," he said to himself. "It is no more!"

He drew in a breath, stopped in the midst of a sigh, stretched out, and died.

(Tolstoy 2003: 152)

References

Aries, Philippe (1974) *Western Attitudes Toward Death.* Johns Hopkins University Press, Baltimore.

Baugher, John Eric (2008) Encountering the intimate stranger. In *The Pulse of Death NOW: The Austin H. Kutscher Memorial Conference.* The Kellog Center, International Affairs Building, Columbia University, NY.

Bedell, Susanna, E., Karen Cadenhead, and Thomas B. Graboys (2001) The Doctor's Letter of Condolence. *New England Journal of Medicine, 344*(15),1162–64.

Block, Susan, D., and Andrew Billings J. (2005) Learning from the Dying. *New England Journal of Medicine, 353*(13), 1313–15.

Campo, R. (2004) Just the Facts. *New England Journal of Medicine, 351*(12), 1167–69.

Charon, R. (2006) *Narrative Medicine: Honoring the Stories of Illness.* Oxford University Press, New York.

Connelly, J. (2002) In the Absence of Narrative. In *Stories Matter: The Role of Narrative in Medical Ethics* (eds. R. Charon and M. Montello). Routledge, NewYork, NY.

DasGupta, Sayantani (2007) Between tillness and story: lessons of children's illness narratives. *Pediatrics, 119*(6), 1384–91.

———. 2008. Narrative humility. *The Lancet, 371,* 980–81.

Frank, Arthur, W. (1995) *The Wounded Storyteller: Body, Illness and Ethics.* University of Chicago Press, Chicago, IL.

———. 2004a. The renewal of generosity: illness, medicine and how to live. University of Chicago Press, Chicago, IL.

———. 2004b. Asking the right questions about pain: narrative and phronesis. *Literature & Medicine, 23*(2), 209–25.

Irvine, Craig, A. (2005) The other side of silence: levinas, medicine, and literature. *Literature & Medicine, 24*(1), 8–18.

———. 2009. The ethics of self-care. In *Faculty Health in Academic Medicine: Physicians, Scientists, and the Pressures of Success,* (eds. T. J. Goodrich, T. R. Cole, and E. R. Gritz). Humana Press, NewYork, NY.

Irvine, P. (1985) The attending at the funeral. *New England Journal of Medicine, 312,* 1704–05.

Kleinman, Arthur (1988) *The Illness Narratives: Suffering, Healing and the Human Condition.* Basic Books, New York, NY.

Laderman, Gary (2003) *Rest in Peace: A Cultural History of Death and the Funeral Home in Twentieth Century America.* Oxford University Press, NewYork, NY.

Morrison, Toni (1993) Nobel Lecture. *Nobel Prize in Literature.* Available at: http://nobelprize.org/nobel_prizes/literature/laureates/1993/morrison-lecture.html.

Phillips, R.D. (2006) *Active Religion's Passive Voice* June 17, 1985 [cited December 8, 2006]. Available at: http://www.uuma.org/BerryStreet/Essays/BSE1985.htm.

Sontag, Susan (1988) *Illness as Metaphor.* Anchor Books, New York.

Tolstoy, Leo (2003) *The Death of Ivan Ilych and Other Stories.* Signet Classic, NewYork, NY.

Chapter 3

Narrative interviews and research

Yasmin Gunaratnam

> For look! Within my hollow hand,
> While round the earth careens,
> I hold a single grain of sand
> And wonder what it means.
> Ah! If I had the eyes to see,
> And brain to understand,
> I think Life's mystery might be
> Solved in this grain of sand
> (*Service*, 1954)

I begin this chapter on narrative research in palliative care with a detour into geo-physics and the discipline of luminescence dating that uses light to date minerals such as quartz (Aitken, 1998). I know little about luminescence dating, but I was drawn into listening to a friend discuss a methodological and theoretical problem he was facing in dating sand grains as a part of wider work on modelling climate change. Individual sand grains store a signal that can be used to date their age (the time at which they were deposited). The signal is released when grains are exposed to light under laboratory conditions. The problem is that signals can be misleading: grains of sand drawn from the same sample can emit different signals.

I have little doubt that what captivated me about this problem was the sheer quantum magic of the vast scales of life inscribed and played out in these minis-cule arena; how grains of sand can illuminate – quite literally – chronotopic truths about how they have been positioned temporally and spatially in our universe. As I listened to the scientist's story, I also saw connections across disciplines and raw materials, between the problems in luminescence dating, and ongoing methodological questions and debates in narrative research, where narratives have been conceptualized as microcosmic 'intimations' of the narrator's origins in and evolving relations to their social universe (Scheff, 1997: 48), complicating notions of inside and outside, then and now.

Let me explain some more: in my understanding, what the luminescence scientist does is to try and interpret the biographical story (signal) of individual grains of sand; sometimes these stories do not express wider events and history accurately. The problem for the scientist is to find ways of interpreting the meaning of these different stories, while also identifying the source of the variations between them. Once there is sufficient information about the causes of such variations, methods can be applied or developed to 'read' the different stories and to treat the grains of sand individually. With these methods, the scientist's analytic pacing between the idiosyncrasies of a single grain and its wider context is more focussed and honed. All in all, the process does not so much produce definitive answers, as refine the research methods and questions, connecting the particular to more general paradigms of knowledge, and bringing closer the unintelligible.

There are limits of course, to the parallels that we can draw between scientific and narrative methods. Nevertheless, the problem of method and interpretation in luminescence dating is a powerful metaphor. What are the relationships between narrative accounts of experience and events? How suitable are the methods that we use in helping us to elicit and interpret narrative accounts? What place/space do we give to the unintelligible, the unsaid, and to the incompleteness of interpretation as necessarily always 'work-in-progress'? And how attuned are our methods to difference and to situation, to narratives as 'chronotopes' providing unique perspectives on time and context?

The literary theorist Bakhtin asserted that 'the chronotope makes narrative events concrete, makes them take on flesh, causes blood to flow in their veins' (1981: 250). If narratives can pulsate with lived life, it is also the case that research methods and analysis can coagulate or sometimes extinguish this life. There is a tendency in narrative research in palliative care to smooth out the inconsistencies and the flux of narrated experience; the moments and places in which experience thickens or thins, when it cannot account for itself in words, or when it turns around and invents something extraordinary. In our attempts at making sense, narrative analysis can become a *post hoc* restoration of rational meaning – a coming 'full circle and ending up facing backwards' (Frosh, 2007: 644). If narrative accounts bewilder us and throw us off course *in situ*, there is the reassuring consolation that all will be revealed in the analysis stages of research.

My own experiences of research tell a different story. In what follows I want to show how I have negotiated (and continue to negotiate) the methodological and ethical path between knowing and not-knowing (Badiou, 2002).

I am especially concerned with how uncertainty in understanding can signify ethical events both in terms of the ethical struggle of the narrator (which has implications for emotional support provided in the research process[1]), but also how analytic uncertainty can mark an opening up to others 'whose difference inspires and moves us' (Diprose, 2002: 191).

In giving specific attention to narrative interviews, I return to the very beginnings of my research with hospice patients through a single case study of Phyllis (a pseudonym). Phyllis was the first patient I interviewed. I have used her stories in teaching and training – but never before for publication. I will re-examine these interviews in the light of my greater and ongoing experience with narrative methods, rewinding to the past, when at the time of the interviews I was unaware of narrative methodology, and fast-forwarding to my present interpretations. By way of introduction, I will outline the basic tenets of narrative interviews. Then, through Phyllis's interviews I will examine assumptions about language and sense-making (subjectivity) that underlie narrative interview methods. In the final sections of the chapter, I point to the limitations of narrative analysis.

Narrative interviews and the interviewer as midwife

When I began my ethnographic research in palliative care over a decade ago, I had intended to conduct semi-structured interviews with migrants who were hospice patients. I was concerned with understanding identity at the end of life and with examining the responsiveness of the holistic care model to social differences. I had developed questions from the research and policy literature that I wanted patients to engage with. After reviewing the first of my five 'pilot' interviews, I realized that my interview schedule was eliciting wide-ranging biographical narratives.

At that time, my predominant concern was with how to interpret and analyse these diverse accounts and their thematic fields. Only after my research had been completed, and through subsequent training in the biographical narrative interpretive method (see Chamberlayne et al. 2000; Wengraf 2001) was I better able to understand how the content and structuring of questions can either facilitate or constrain the life of narratives. I now see the role of the researcher and/or practitioner as a midwife to narrative, with her questions and attentiveness skilfully helping or coaxing a narrative into the world (see also DasGupta, Irvine and Spiegel this volume), by encouraging and supporting deeper recall and a 'being-there' experiencing.

At a basic level, what I have learned is that to elicit narrative you need to ask narrative-inducing questions; these are questions that ask about events: open, 'what happened?' type questions, rather than questions that ask for opinion, rationalization, or generalization. This is because opinions and rationalizations can be constrained by what is felt to be socially acceptable or desirable (Goffman, 1968); they are often pre-formulated and rehearsed, providing insight into autobiographical theory but remaining somewhat distant from experience.

A related point concerns the interview relationship and a non-directive attentiveness on the part of the interviewer. As my interviews with Phyllis will reveal, apparently unrelated narratives can express a submerged connectedness of experience in which the meaning frameworks surrounding topics can be unknowable for both researchers and research participants (Hollway and Jefferson, 2000a). This is one reason why some narrative interview methods are designed around asking one broad narrative-inducing question (see Riemann, 2003), with subsequent questions being framed by this initial narrative and following strictly the order of the topics freely associated by the narrator. The rationale being that this initial narrative has a shape or 'gestalt' of sedimented experience that is a part of a unique system of relevance. One of the most challenging, but vital skills for a narrative researcher/midwife is to 'go with the flow'; to allow the gestalt to emerge in its own way – and without interruptions – no matter how incoherent or 'off the point' certain accounts can feel.

I will examine the apparent disjointedness of narratives further in my discussion of Phyllis's interviews. I will also identify more specifically, what I see as the insufficiency of some common assumptions and practices in qualitative interviews.

Phyllis

Phyllis was an Anglo-Indian woman in her sixties. In the first stages of our interview, Phyllis told me that she avoided talk about death and dying; she confronted and disparaged others such as a neighbour who had talked about dying, and she attempted to carry on with household chores even when they were becoming increasingly unmanageable, because 'I like to do all the things that I was doing before.' Phyllis limited her contact with the hospice, (describing how 'it gives me the creeps') because of its associations with death.

Phyllis lived with her older sister and widowed mother in their owner-occupied house, in an affluent, suburban area. She saw herself as the 'the sole get-up-and-go person in the house', competent in home economics, a dancer and socialite, who took great pride in her glamorous appearance. During our first interview, I was aware of Phyllis's sister moving about in another part of the house. My field notes describe how 'Phyllis took charge of the interview from the beginning', a reference to my feelings that the interview had veered away from my topic guide. Indeed, Phyllis was a forceful presence and a skilled and practised narrator. Many of her narratives felt well-worn, a quality that was confirmed by her frequent reference to other people's responses to the narratives that she recounted.

Towards the beginning of the first interview, Phyllis told me that since the diagnosis of her breast cancer she had avoided reading the newspapers and would switch off the television whenever there was any reporting of death-related incidents. She said:

> I hate to even think when it's going to happen (her death). So I don't like to discuss it.... I talk about everything, but I never bring this thing up.... I don't want to know, because at the back of my mind I am praying very hard and taking each day as it comes.

By telling me about her avoidance of death-related words and subjects at the beginning of each of our two interviews, we can see something of the dialogic quality of interviews in which the 'interviewer and interviewee negotiate some degree of agreement on what they will talk about, and how' (Mishler, 1999: xvi). The transcript of the interview shows that I did not ask any questions relating to the progression of Phyllis's breast cancer that had spread to her lungs. In retrospect, it also felt that Phyllis used this first interview to 'test me out' at different levels and to see how I took account of her need to avoid talking about death and dying.

Aspects of this testing-out/trust-building process can be seen in how Phyllis questioned me about my own ethnicity and religion at the end of our first interview, when the tape recorder had been packed away. My fieldnotes – written on the day of the interview – record that I had felt anxious when Phyllis had asked these questions because she had made repeated references to the importance of her Catholic religion, although she had also talked about changes in her religious practice since the reoccurrence of her cancer: 'I've always been a fervent believer of my prayer . . . but I can't pray as I was before, because my mind's not focusing very well. My mind is er (2) troubled . . . I feel "How can this have happened to me? What did I do wrong?"

I had been brought up as a Catholic but I am not religious, and I had been anxious about whether this difference could have negative effects upon our research relationship and upon what Phyllis would feel able to tell me. In the event I told Phyllis about my Catholic background and that I was no longer religious. As I gathered my things to leave, Phyllis told me that she had 'troubles' on her mind that she wanted to talk about at the next interview.

Troubles

At our second interview, a month later, Phyllis's sister and mother were not at home, but her brother, who was visiting from East Africa, was in another part of the house for about the first 20 minutes of the interview. During this time, Phyllis spoke more about her reluctance to go to the hospice. In response to a question from me about whether she had 'had a look around the hospice at all?', she talked about why she did not want to go to the hospice day centre ('that's the end of the world for me'), linking this to a story about a friend's recent death. It was through this latter narrative that Phyllis came to the 'troubles' that she had mentioned previously:

> Don't forget I just lost my friend in August who died of ovarian cancer, and I took it to heart. She was my ex-boyfriend's sister. I've known her since 1969.... August the 18th she died and the end of September I was ill, and I'm sure it was all the shock. My mum didn't want me to go and see her in the church. But her husband said to me 'Look Phil, we're bringing the body to the church for half an hour, so if you want to see your friend for the last time, who's to stop you?' Because my ex-boyfriend is married (whispered), and we had a, I've been with him for so many years you know, and I was heartbroken as well, and I still feel that same about him. That was the thing I was telling you.

Most of our second interview was taken up with this 30-year, intermittent affair. At the point when Phyllis first told me about the relationship, I abandoned my topic guide, as Phyllis talked in detail about her dilemmas about both wanting to end the relationship, but also continuing to see and love the unnamed man – the husband of a friend. Given my identification as an unknown South-Asian woman from a Catholic background, Phyllis's own ethno-religious identity, and the fact that her brother was in the house at this point of the interview, Phyllis's account of her relationship would appear to involve multiple areas of difficulty and threat.

In broad terms, the public status of older Anglo-Indian, Catholic women, particularly those in the middle classes, is related to sexual morality. To have a long-term affair, with the husband of a friend, would have been in direct contravention of cultural and religious norms. These transgressions would have brought with them the danger of being ostracized both from family and from the wider Anglo-Indian networks – which were a significant part of Phyllis's life – together with more personal costs such as those arising from feelings of guilt, shame, anger and resentment. Clues to such emotions can be found by examining and categorizing changes in the way an account is narrated (known as a 'textsort change', Wengraf, 2001). For instance, it is notable that in talking about this relationship, Phyllis moved away from description and narration and into argumentation and evaluation, suggesting a need to defend and/or justify herself.

If this relationship was potentially a difficult and threatening topic for Phyllis to talk about, then what is particularly surprising is that it was also through her stories of the affair that Phyllis was able to talk about the prospect of her death.

She did this, indirectly at first, making connections between her inability to end the relationship and her inability to come to terms with her own death:

> But I should just put it (the relationship) to the back of my mind really. It's not going to get me anywhere. But I can't come to grips, like I can't come to grips with my (2), me popping off with cancer. I can't come to grips with me not (1) ever being away from this guy for long.

In the narrative connections between the relationship and the prospect of her death from cancer were hesitant tensions between knowing and not-knowing. Such tensions can be read into the uncharacteristic pauses (noted and timed in seconds in brackets in the excerpt above) that follow both of Phyllis's pronouncements about 'coming to grips with'. Within and through the interview process, Phyllis was able to move between different levels of narrated knowledge and awareness and inhabit more than one position, enabling a greater ambivalence to be expressed; an ambivalence that is evoked in her use of a double negative ('I can't come to grips with me not (1) ever being away from this guy for long') that suggests that she has, despite her own efforts, faced this unbearable known.

Narrative connections

In abandoning my topic guide at the point when Phyllis told me about the relationship, my role in the second interview now reads like a stumbling and improvized mixture of clarifying and reflecting back the themes in Phyllis's accounts. I remember feeling anxious and unsure about how to proceed with the interview. Part of this anxiety sprang – and continues to spring – from a culturally related sense of unease and jeopardy in talking (and now writing) openly about the affair with an older woman, who outside of the interview relationship I would usually defer to as an 'aunty'. Sayantani DasGupta (1999) has written of similar dynamics in her medical training when she had to question a grandmother about sex. She describes how 'I gulped inwardly, trying to swallow the ominous feeling that the long hand of my own Granny would appear, at any minute, around the globe from India to slap her impudent granddaughter . . . it was me who was red-faced at the cultural impropriety of asking a grandmother to tell me about her sex life' (p. 138).

It is significant that the transcript shows that I moved far away from narrative-inducing 'what happened?' style questions in this part of the interview. The shape of the transcript here is also different from the rest of the interview and from my first interview with Phyllis. As an indicator of whether an interview is a narrative interview or not, in the very first stages of analysis, I now look at the shape of the interview transcript. In general, narrative interviews are characterized by long stretches of talk from the research participant, unbroken by questions or interjections from the interviewer. Following Phyllis's initial disclosure about the affair, the transcript became more fissured and spiky.

Although this was a non-narrative inducing interview style, it took place after narrative had been elicited, and in response to the content of Phyllis's narrative about the affair. This reflecting back of narrative themes had the effect of drawing out more tentative connections, a claim that can be assessed with regard to the next extract (that followed on closely from the previous one). Here, my articulation of the implicit links between the affair and Phyllis's illness provoked further reflection from Phyllis about the delicate relationships between her outer and inner worlds; between avoidance and self-awareness and knowledge:

> Yasmin: So do you want to know one way or the other (about the relationship)?
>
> Phyllis: Umm. But, how to know it? I know. I know the answer, just like I know about my cancer. I know what the answer's going to be here and I can't bear to face it.
>
> Yasmin: That's interesting because you've made two, two (1) examples there before when you said –
>
> Phyllis: Which is so identical.
>
> Yasmin: Yeah, how you're dealing with your illness is quite similar to how you're dealing with him –
>
> Phyllis: Yes. It's terminal there. It's terminal here. I mean if you go to see, you use the word terminal here you can use the same here as well, although it doesn't fit very well in this category . . .

What is striking about this extract is Phyllis's freely associated use of the unambiguous word 'terminal', which came out so quickly that it surprised us both. It was an utterance, spoken with harsh economy, that presented 'trouble' for Phyllis's previous investment in unfolding future possibilities, and she attempts to repair this dissonance by immediately questioning the fit of the word 'terminal'. However fleeting and accidental this utterance appears, it shifted something in the interview. Phyllis's account became more nuanced, and for the first time opened out towards moral questions: 'He was already married . . . which I shouldn't have carried on'. In recycling a popular discourse that in some cases, married men can leave their families for their lover, Phyllis undermined this discourse with something closely evocative of annihilation: 'But then on the other hand being with you, he can destroy you as well. So it's a gamble.' Travelling the emotional lines of connection between her illness and the impossible relationship, Phyllis arrived in an entirely different place:

> See I don't want to hear it?. . . . That same feeling like the illness. I don't want to hear about my illness. If I get bad then I will be first one to know it myself, that that's the end for me.

As Arthur Frank (Chapter 10) has recognized, stories can function to help people regain a sense of agency and responsibility in their lives. This can happen when stories make connections – both in terms of the correspondences made and felt by the narrator, and in the relationship between the narrator and listener. For Frank, it is the offered 'presence' of the listener as a witness to another's suffering that is connective. This is in essence a moral point. Looked at through a methodological lens it suggests the value of openness and passivity on the part of the researcher. As Jones (2003: 60) reminds us, 'The turn to narrative inquiry shifts the role of the researcher from being a knowledge-privileged investigator to a reflective passive participant during the storytelling process.'

Theory and narrative interviews

While staying with the specificities of Phyllis's narratives, I want to return to questions of methodology and theory that underlie narrative interviewing. As a novice narrative interviewer at the time, I moved between an 'irritating mix' (Riemann, 2003) of questions that asked, unsystematically, for narrative and opinions; a common practice in qualitative interviewing, and one which has implications for the types of account that are generated. It is not so much that narrative interviewers never ask questions involving opinion and evaluation, it is more that such questions should ideally be asked after the research participant has freely given and completed their initial, uninterrupted narrative about experienced events.

The rationale behind the focus upon questions that ask about experiences and events is related to assumptions about language and subjectivity. Many interview methods are based upon notions of language as a transparent representation of internal and external states, assuming a research subject that 'one can ask questions and get straight answers, one that knows its own mind and can communicate this in a largely autonomous fashion' (Hollway, 2001:13). In narrative research however, we are cautious about the transparency of language. Language is performative, and narrated accounts 'do things' (see Paley and Eva this volume). Accounts can show us or conceal aspects of the identity or actions of the teller (Gunaratnam, 2003); they circulate and question social values and beliefs (Billig, et al. 1988); they involve conscious and unconscious emotions (Hollway and Jefferson, 2000a); and through the act of narration they affect both the narrator and the listener (Frosh, 2007).

Language and subjectivity

In my research I find that I move between four main approaches to language: I take language as representing events that have happened; as communicating the non-rational and emotional; as producing experience; and as bringing people into ethical relationships.

I most often take language as being literal when it is used to convey external 'facts'; those bare descriptions of events, people, or things that could be verified with reference to documentary data: Phyllis migrated to the United Kingdom in 1969; she was first diagnosed with breast cancer in 1993. My approach to narratives as containing non-rational and involuntary expression in which emotions, particularly those that are painful or difficult, can be hidden or avoided has been informed by psychoanalysis – a discipline that is concerned with the workings of the unconscious mind. Psychoanalytically inspired approaches to narrative are varied, ranging from perspectives that seek to uncover the deep order and structure of the unconscious (Klein, 1975), to those that view the unconscious mind as an emergent and inter-relational process without pre-existing form (Lacan, 1973). At a general level, I have found psychoanalytic concepts valuable in attending to what Clarke (2006: 1161) describes as 'the mad, often crazy side of our lives' – such as those aspects of narrative that appear contradictory and unintentional. Recognition of involuntary expression through narrative has led some authors to suggest that narrators are always 'motivated not to know certain aspects of themselves and . . . produce accounts which avoid such knowledge' (Hollway and Jefferson, 2000b: 169). Significantly, as Tom Wengraf (2000) has pointed out, the researcher can also be motivated not to recognize certain things, and such defensive not-knowing can intrude into the interviewing, data analysis and writing up stages of research. Although such defensiveness cannot be eliminated, Wengraf suggests that it can be identified and combated by forms of analytic group work, in which the diversity – and I would add the autonomy of the analysis group from the research project – is important.

My recognition of narrative and stories as conveying and *doing* unconscious emotions has been supplemented with ideas from discursive psychology, and more specifically 'discourse analysis' (Potter and Wetherell, 1987). From a discourse analytic, language does not so much represent reality, it produces and shapes it. So, rather than narratives being seen as accurate reports of internal states or external 'facts', in discourse analysis talk and narrative are conceptualized as a form of social action (Wilkinson and Kitzinger, 2000), 'intensely located' in their specific interactional contexts and a part of the ongoing identity work of speakers (Wetherell and Edley, 1998: 170). For example, in focus groups with women with breast cancer, Wilkinson and Kitzinger (2000) used discourse analysis to examine talk about 'thinking positive'. By examining how women used the phrase 'thinking positive' in talking to each other, Wilkinson and Kitzinger found that 'thinking positive' functioned as a cultural idiom, serving to minimize the interactional impact of difficult experiences and emotions so that 'the speaker can bring her troubles talk to an "upbeat" end, relieving her listeners of a potential conversational burden' (p. 805).

One does not have to subscribe to either psychoanalysis or discourse analysis to recognize how narratives and stories can be shaped by the emotional and the social. Nonetheless, the point is that our interviewing and/or consulting practices are not neutral or benign – every single time that we elicit and interpret a narrative we are drawing upon (usually implicit) assumptions about language and subjectivity. Explicating these assumptions is a definitive feature of reflective practice (see Forbes, this volume) and what is known as 'reflexivity' in social science research. Reflexivity involves a critical stance to existing concepts and research methods, recognizing that these are not objective and value free, but are influenced by the social context – so that they both affect and produce what we come to know.

Reflexive/reflective practice also strives to recognize how our social and biographical experiences are a part of what is often referred to as the 'co-production' of narratives, and critical attention has been given to the researcher's emotional responses, particularly in examining ethics. As Riessman (2005: 473) has suggested: 'The investigator's emotions are highly relevant to conversations about ethics because emotions do moral work: they embody judgments about value.' Practices that support reflexivity include the use of field notes in analysis that record interview dynamics (see Wengraf, 2001); regular fieldwork supervision sessions that interrogate research relationships and provide a forum where researchers can bring their own 'troubles' and emotions; and group analysis of data to encourage multiple perspectives.

Yet, no matter how rigorous our research methods and practices are, narrative analysis is always partial and provisional. It is this recognition that brings me to my fourth approach to language: language as ethics. The psychologist Stephen Frosh (2007) has pointed out that experience always exceeds narrative (and, of course, *vice versa*). This is not only because experience is itself multifarious and multi-sensual, not simply because there are many ways of narrating the same events, but also because to narrate an experience is to change it – and to change it in relation to another. For Frosh, 'The speaking of the thing acts as a wager, a point at which something is risked into existence' (p. 641); an ethical model of relating that Frosh derives from the work of the feminist philosopher, Judith Butler:

> To ask for recognition, or to offer it, is precisely not to ask for recognition for what one already is. It is to solicit a becoming, to instigate a transformation, to petition the future always in relation to the Other.
>
> (Butler, 2004: 25)

In Frosh's view, one way of preserving the multiplicity and relationality of narratives is to pursue an analysis that holds on to 'disrupting and disorganising' interpretations; analysis that refuses the drive towards the cleaning-up and pulling-together impulses of the researcher/practitioner in seeking out the unifying story-line/s that can summarize a narrated life.

Of course, in 'real-word' research and professional practice we are bound to the pinning down of interpretation. It is not difficult for me to imagine Phyllis's hospice nurse at a start-of-day multidisciplinary team meeting introducing Phyllis as a 'complicated and anxious lady' and for elements of Phyllis's 'death denial' and the affair, to have real value and relevance, for example, in attempts (that were made) to open-up conversations with Phyllis about her death and future care planning. The reality is that not many of us would want practitioners who, full of angst about preserving multiplicity, avoid interpretation and become lost in our narrative complexity. While the drive towards the production of narrative coherence may have had its day (Mishler, 1999), developments in areas such as narrative medicine are providing valuable insights into working with, rather than against, the incompleteness and mysteries of narrative experience (see also Stanworth, this volume). The message is that full understanding and narrative coherence is not necessary to accompany people through profoundly difficult and confusing times (Charon, 2006).

The art of not-knowing

In the preceding discussion, I have wanted to show and respect the value of some of the guiding principles of narrative interview methods, while also using my interviews with Phyllis to reflect the difficulties of what Lather (2001: 205) refers to as 'the nostalgic desire for immediacy and transparency of reference' that 'strikes the epistemological paradox of . . . knowing both too little and too much'. There is no doubt that my interviews with Phyllis gave me more than I could ever have expected. Phyllis was not the 'typical' Anglo-Indian, Catholic 'other-woman' full of remorse about her illicit relationship, particularly when faced with her death ('I loved every minute of it'). She pushed to the limits the hospice narrative of 'living until you die', pioneering her own version of a 'good death' by keeping her options open. And in this way her narratives also resonate with existing questions about the valorizing of open-awareness of dying as a historical and Northern European invention.

Such knowledge, is however, tempered by the complexity that organized Phyllis's stories; for while she narrated herself into many conventional plot lines (woman as victim, death-denying/stoical older patient), these narrations always had a twist, subverting what they appeared to repeat, and holding open interpretation. And although Phyllis's accounts of the affair provide some biographical clues into her idiosyncratic investments in living with disturbing external realities, it is the endless deferrals, an irreverent gambling with the future, and the tension between knowing and not-knowing that I am left with. While certain stories may be organized around and build towards revelation and purposeful resolution (see Chapter 1), lives are not always lived or died in this way.

Such irresolution in interpretation is far from unique. I believe that narrative practitioners are acutely aware of what exceeds and escapes technique and knowledge, and this is an integral, though under-discussed part of the challenges and the ethics of narrative-based practice. It is also how others make their mark upon us, how 'the skin that holds our self-possession is broken; we cannot tell the difference between what touches and what is touched' (Diprose, 2002: 191). This is not to shy away from interpretation or to devalue narrative scholarship that has generated significant insights into the effects of narrative and the strange little ways that we tell ourselves (and are told) into being. But I am not sure that the answer lies wholly in better conceptualization, methodology, or technique.

The gaps and questions in my research in palliative care have led me to other disciplines and forms of representation, particularly art[2] that more freely admits and expresses incoherence (Gunaratnam, 2007) and through which I can better express and honour the ways in which research participants have made impressions upon me – how words, images, and places from interviews flash into my consciousness, how I often feel the presence of those who have died, and how new possibilities emerge continually from narrated accounts.

The fundamental problematic of interpretation, regardless of discipline, is that it is always a risky, emotion-laden and ethical business. And for me, the chains of association between a scientist working in a laboratory with sand grains and a narrative practitioner, lie in how we might practise our respective crafts in ways that aspire to the honing of technique and skill and that give recognition to our being touched (Diprose, 2002), while all the time remaining faithful and vulnerable to the unknown (Badiou, 2002).

Notes

1. In the research reported here I ensured that research participants were aware that they could talk further about issues that arose in the interviews with trained professionals at the hospice and at independent organizations.
2. I have written two poems inspired by Phyllis (Gunaratnam, 2008).

References

Aitken, M. (1998) *An Introduction to Optical Dating*. Oxford University Press, Oxford.
Badiou, A. (2002) *Ethics – An Essay on the Understanding of Evil*. Verso, London.

Bakhtin, M. M. (1981). *The Dialogic Imagination: Four Essays*. University of Texas Press, Austin TX.

Billig, M., Condor, S., Edwards, D., Gane, M., Middleton, D., and Radley, A. (1988) *Ideological Dilemmas: A Social Psychology of Everyday Thinking*. Sage, London.

Butler, J. (2004). *Precarious Life*. Verso, London.

Chamberlayne, P., Bornat, J., and Wengraf, T. (2000) (eds) *The Turn to Biographical Methods in Social Science: Comparative Issues and Examples*. Routledge, London.

Charon, R. (2006) *Narrative Medicine – Honoring the Stories of Illness*. Oxford University Press, Oxford.

Clarke, S. (2006) Theory and practice: psychoanalytic sociology as psycho-social studies. *Sociology*, **40**(6), 1153–69.

DasGupta, S. (1999) *Her Own Medicine: A Woman's Journey From Student to Doctor*. Ballantine, New York.

Diprose, R. (2002) *Corporeal Generosity – On Giving Nietzche, Merleau-Ponty and Levinas*. State University of New York Press, New York.

Frosh, S. (2007) Disintegrating qualitative research. *Theory and Psychology*, **17**, 635–53.

Goffman, E. (1968). *Asylums. Essays on the Social Situation of Mental Patients and Other Inmates*. Harmondsworth, Penguin, UK.

Gunaratnam, Y. (2003) *Researching Race and Ethnicity: Methods, Knowledge and Power*. Sage, London.

Gunaratnam, Y. (2007) Where is the love? Art, aesthetics and research. *Journal of Social Work Practice*, **21**(3), 271–87.

Gunaratnam, Y. (2008) For Phyllis; and blind date. In *Making Sense of Death, Dying and Bereavement: An Anthology* (eds. C. Bartholomew and S. Earle). Sage, London. pp. 44–6.

Hollway, W. (2001) The psycho-social subject in 'evidence-based' practice. *Journal of Social Work Practice*, **15**(1), 9–22.

Hollway, W. and Jefferson, T. (2000a) *Doing Qualitative Research Differently, Free Association, Narrative and the Interview Method*. Sage, London.

Hollway, W. and Jefferson, T. (2000b) Biography, anxiety and the experience of locality. In *The Turn to Biographical Methods in Social Science: Comparative Issues and Examples* (eds. P. Chamberlayne, J. Bornat, and T. Wengraf). Routledge, London. pp. 167–80.

Jones, K. (2003) The turn to a narrative knowing of persons: one method explored. *Nursing Times Research*, **8**(1), 60–71.

Klein, M. (1975) *Love, Guilt and Reparation and Other Works 1921–1945*. Hogarth Press Ltd, London.

Lacan, J. (1973) *The Four Fundamental Concepts of Psychoanalysis*. Penguin, Harmondsworth.

Lather, P. (2001) Postbook: working the ruins of feminist ethnography. *Signs*, **27**(1), 199–227.

Mishler, E. (1999) *Storylines: Craftartists' Narratives of Identity*. Harvard University Press, Cambridge, MA and London.

Potter, J. and Wetherell, M. (1987) *Discourse and Social Psychology*. Sage, London.

Riemann, G. (2003, September). A joint project against the backdrop of a research tradition: an introduction to "Doing Biographical Research" [36 paragraphs]. *Forum Qualitative Sozialforschung / Forum: Qualitative Social Research* [Online Journal], 4(3),

Art. 18. Available at: http://www.qualitative-research.net/fqs-texte/ 3-03/3-03hrsg-e.htm Retrieved May 2008.

Riessman, C. (2005) Exporting ethics: a narrative about narrative research in South India. *Health*, **9**(4), 473–90.

Scheff, T. (1997) *Emotions, the Social Bond, and Human Reality: Part/Whole Analysis.* Cambridge University Press, Cambridge.

Service, R. (1954) A grain of sand. In *Carols of an Old Codger*. Dodd Mead, New York.

Wengraf, T. (2000) Uncovering the general from within the particular: from Contingencies to typologies in the understanding of cases. In *The Turn to Biographical Methods in Social Science: Comparative Issues and Examples* (eds. P. Chamberlayne, J. Bornat, and T. Wengraf). Routledge, London. pp. 140–64.

Wengraf, T. (2001) *Qualitative Research Interviewing. Biographic Narrative and Semi-structured Method.* Sage, London.

Wetherell, M. and Edley, N. (1998) Gender practices: steps in the analysis of men and masculinities. In *Standpoints and Differences: Essays in the Practice of Feminist Psychology* (eds. K. Henwood, C. Griffin, and A. Phoenix). Sage, London, pp. 165–73.

Wilkinson, S. and Kitzinger, C. (2000) Thinking Differently About Thinking Positive: A discursive approach to cancer patients' talk. *Social Science & Medicine*, **50**, 797–811.

Chapter 4

Narrative-based evidence in palliative care

Kim Devery

Evidence and 'evidence-based practice' are terms with an increasingly high profile in health and social care. Evidence is the medium which provides proof that a health intervention works well. Specific interventions, such as medications and particular communication approaches, require confirmation of efficiency. This confirmation can minimize wasteful, futile, or even harmful interventions.

Evidence and 'evidence-based practice' are also terms that can, and have, provoked considerable debate and angst. Many have questioned just what type of evidence should provide proof of quality. Clinician Archie Cochrane (1972) and clinical epidemiologist David Sackett (1996) proposed that evidence should change to include population-based knowledge generated from specific types of research. Prior to the 1970s, evidence generated from clinical experience and medical sciences had underscored the main theoretical understandings for medical knowledge (Timmermans and Berg, 2003).

The social psychologist Wendy Hollway (2001) describes how the phrase 'evidence-based practice' crept up on her, accruing gradual, intuitive meanings in her imagination. As someone concerned with how care can be responsive to the complexities, diversity, and singularity of human experience, she felt initially that 'evidence-based practice' negated the role of learning from experience in professional practice, while also threatening to 'impose reductive and standardised interventions' (p.10). The physician and pioneer of narrative-based medicine in the United Kingdom, Trisha Greenhalgh (2004) found huge gaps between the ideal of systematic reviews used in evidence-based research, and research that informs policy-making. In examining the research literature, Greenhalgh found that the line between 'science' and 'values' was hazy in research, and that the research reviews that had impacted upon policy were those that 'break all the fundamental rules of systematic reviewing' (p.352). Greenhalgh and her team went on to propose a 'meta-narrative mapping' approach, where key characteristics of narrative such as time, emplotment, and meaning-making were used to make sense of the evidence of research findings. In palliative care, more recent discussions (Aoun and Krisjanson, 2005; Devery, 2006) have held out a fundamental challenge: how, given palliative care's commitment to personalized, holistic care, and multidisciplinary team working, might the specialty develop and value evidence frameworks beyond evidence-based medicine's 'gold standard' of randomized controlled trials (RCT)?

In this chapter, I will examine the potential of narrative as evidence in palliative care. That is, how knowledge derived from narratives and stories might be used to broaden (or perhaps re-validate) the evidence base of palliative care in order to inform families and patients, professionals, health and social care services, communities, and policy-makers. The basis of my argument is that a wide variety of knowledge, and evidence of it, is needed in palliative care: we need to know about the efficacy of therapeutic interventions, self-care, the experience and meaning of illness and symptoms (see Bolton and Koffman, this volume), communication with patients and families, and much more.

A key theme in my discussion will be the importance of human judgement in the interpretation and application of evidence. For example, while 'instrumental knowledge' (Aoun and Kristjanson, 2005: 464) developed through traditional scientific approaches such as RCT's often appears to be the basis that informs the prescription of pain-relieving drugs, it is judgement derived from a combination of knowledge, experience, and values (in combination with what the patient/family wants) that will inform what is prescribed, how, and when. Other forms of knowledge will be needed to guide a practitioner in the care given to a patient who says that she does not need rehabilitative support because she is well organized and 'coping' (see Eva, this volume).

In what follows, I discuss the rationale behind evidence-based medicine and briefly describe randomized control trials. I then move on to look at evidence in palliative care and suggest what form narrative-based evidence in palliative care might take.

Evidence-based medicine

A widely used definition of evidence-based medicine is:

> the conscientious, explicit, and judicious use of current best evidence in making decisions about the care of individual patients. The practice of evidence-based medicine means integrating individual clinical expertise with the best available external clinical evidence from systematic research.
>
> (Sackett et al. 1996: 71)

"External clinical evidence" in this context refers to population-based and basic scientific research. In 1995, Sackett and Roseberg, supporters of the movement, summarized evidence-based medicine and evidence as:

1. . . . clinical and other health care decisions should be based on the best patient- and population-based as well as laboratory-based evidence;
2. . . . the problem determines the nature and source of evidence to be sought, rather than our habits, protocols or traditions; . . .
3. . . . best evidence calls for the integration of epidemiological and biostatistical ways of thinking with those derived from pathophysiology and our personal experience. . .
4. . . . that the conclusions of this search and critical appraisal of evidence are worthwhile only if they are translated into actions that affect our patients; . . .
5. . . . we should continuously evaluate our performance in applying these ideas.

(Sackett and Roseberg, 1995: 621–2)

How does the practitioner know what is best evidence when reading a research article? And how can the researcher know the best research to design within the framework of evidence-based medicine? A ranking of the types of proof or evidence aims to guide users and producers of research to the definitions of best evidence. Several of these rankings exist and most are fairly similar, see for example the Centre for Evidence-based Medicine Levels of Evidence, Oxford, United Kingdom (May 2001), or the Australian National Health and Medical Research Council (2008). Ultimately, in these rankings, the randomized controlled trial is viewed as the best design of research that yields the strongest evidence:

Study Design (evidence from the best studies available; ranked in descending order of strength)

1. Evidence obtained from randomized controlled trials
2. Evidence obtained from nonrandomized controlled trials.
3. Evidence obtained from cohort or case-control studies.
4. Evidence from ecologic and descriptive studies (e.g. international patterns studies, time series).
5. Opinions of respected authorities based on clinical experience, descriptive studies, or reports of expert committees.

(National Cancer Institute, 2004)

Clearly, in the current climate, not all evidence is viewed as equally convincing or valid. One of the central ideas of evidence-based medicine is that knowledge or evidence systematically generated from patient populations is superior to knowledge generated from clinical experience. However, even proponents of the evidence-based movement admit that there is no evidence to back this belief in the supremacy of systematic population-based research over other types of evidence (Haynes, 2002). Opinions from expert practitioners regarding best patient care are viewed as more fallible than what are seen as 'objective' data generated from systematic research and experimentation (Haynes, 2002). Indeed 'habits, protocol and traditions' have the lowest place in the scheme of the evidence-based movement where the strongest form of evidence is derived from the randomized controlled trial.

What the Randomized Controlled Trial offers

Randomization minimizes the risk of allocation bias, that is, the risk that a patient group in a trial has any advantage in outcome measurement (Jadad and Rennie, 1998). In its simplest form a randomized controlled trial allocates patients or clusters of patients into different groups to receive two or more different interventions. Intervention may be an experimental drug, a placebo, or an usual treatment. Randomization can be achieved by tossing a coin or by following a computer-generated allocation; importantly the participant, the family, health care professionals or researchers do not have any say as to which group the participant is destined.

The creation of the study groups as equal or homogenous as possible is an important feature of the randomized controlled trial, as the effects of the intervention can be understood more clearly. This is often referred to as *internal validity*. Such strength is also a potential weakness however. No matter how well designed the randomized controlled trial or resulting clinical practice guidelines, results always need to be extrapolated for clinical use to an individual patient; that is, in implementing evidence in everyday care, practitioners need to use their judgement in moving between the uniqueness of the patient in front of them with a particular clinical problem and the current evidence generated from homogenous populations (McAlister, et al. 2007; Rothwell, 2005).

In palliative care research, quantitative, comparative, and randomized research collated in the form of a systematic review has shed light on the efficacy of the use of opioids for the symptomatic relief of breathlessness at the end of life (Jennings, et al. 2001).

In the research reviewed, patients (diagnosed with cancer, chronic obstructive pulmonary disease, chronic heart failure, and other advanced lung diseases) were randomized into receiving an opioid (either nebulized, oral, or parental) or placebo, thus mixing the countless other variables that, if otherwise clustered in one group, could have impacted on the outcome measurement. As breathlessness is also a subjective experience, primary outcome measures included how patients reported their experiences of breathlessness using both verbal and visual scales that categorized their responses.

In conclusion, there was no statistically significant difference, in terms of subjective report of breathlessness, in the nebulized morphine group compared to the placebo group (Jennings, et al. 2001). However, there was strong statistical difference between the oral/parental morphine groups and placebo. Those patients who had received either oral or parental morphine reported less breathlessness. Within such an account of research which investigated causal events (e.g. between a particular therapeutic intervention and the symptom of breathlessness) the message for clinicians in planning and prescribing care for the common and distressing symptom of breathlessness is clear.

Evidence in palliative care

However, not all clinical issues in palliative care can be approached in the same manner as a single symptom and not every problem is answered well by randomized controlled trials.

Providing health care to those who are aware of their mortality, who may be in crisis or dying soon raises profound clinical, psycho-social, and ethical challenges for professional practice. A wide variety of knowledge, with supporting evidence, is necessary to equip practitioners to do their job well in palliative care and to therapeutically connect clinician with patient – knowing which drugs to use when, knowing how to communicate with patients about prognosis, knowing how to work well within multidisciplinary teams, understanding what is an appropriate response to difficult ethical situations, and knowing the trajectory of specific diseases. Judgement is the fulcrum on which we lever each other to the view that something is worthy of reliable knowledge or can be seen as 'evidence'. Evidence must satisfy those working in a discipline that certain forms of knowledge are dependable and credible – something *worth* knowing and acting upon.

Considering the extremely broad and complicated nature of knowledge required by professionals to deliver palliative care it is unlikely that one method of research or one type of knowledge (qualitative or quantitative, narrative or numerical) would be adequate to answer all questions.

Think about the clinical issue of communicating with patients about prognosis. Stephen Jay Gould, evolutionary biologist, writes of his own story of prognosis, involving a personal brush with mortality when diagnosed with a type of mesothelioma (see Gould 1991 in Greenhalgh and Hurwitz, 1998: 29–33). Unable to get an answer from his doctor about the course of his illness, he searched the literature to find out more. Within a short time he realized why his doctor had taken, (what he terms), a 'humane' approach by skirting his question. His prognosis was poor – a median mortality of 8 months. He writes:

> Hence the dilemma for humane doctors: since attitude matters so critically, should such a sombre conclusion be advertised, especially since so few people have sufficient

understanding of statistics to evaluate what the statements actually mean? From years
of experience with the small-scale evolution of the Bahamian land snails treated
quantitatively, I have developed this technical knowledge – and I am convinced that it
played a major role in saving my life. Knowledge is indeed power. . .

(Gould, 1991: 475)

Rather than viewing the statistical abstraction of the median as a death
sentence, Gould knew that variation from the average or central tendency was
the way that this statistic operates. He placed himself imaginatively in the half
of those people with this type of illness who live longer than 8 months and was
lucky enough to receive a, then, novel chemotherapy. He outlived his prognosis
by years and his hope was to be one of the new cohort of survivors that
constructed a revised distribution of central tendency.

Stephen Jay Gould's story suggests two things of relevance to this chapter.
First, it brings into sharp focus with a critical bent, how a person feels to hear
a prognosis. Initially crushed by the news, Gould drew upon his own knowledge and expertise to logically unravel what the statistic meant to him as an
individual. This was a task for which he was aptly suited, unlike many other
patients in his position. One can surmize from reading this piece that patients
interpret statistics in various ways, depending on their own worldview. In
addition, it highlights to a clinician the limitations of particular answers one
could offer to patient questions, where statistics about survival make up the
bulk of that answer and where feelings and *attitudes matter so critically*.
Diagnosed in 1982, Gould died in 2002.

Types of evidence

Professionals delivering palliative care use different types of evidence every
day. Consider the patient who is newly admitted to a service; the following
types of knowledge, as a matter of course, would be considered:

1. Patient's story or viewpoint: for example, 'I can't get my breath.'
2. Clinician's standardized observation: for example, auscultation, palpation, history
3. Laboratory test and results: for example, last full blood count, bone scan, CXR
4. Aggregated numerical and statistical data: for example, disease trajectory and
   survival pattern for this patient population.

Evidence of the best intervention is dependent on the particular clinical and
psycho-social situation of a particular patient. Nevertheless, understanding the
patient experience of illness through narrative and excellent communication
and listening will alone not be enough in achieving optimum care.

There are considerable differences for instance between a patient with a pulmonary embolism in urgent physical crisis, and a patient with a more existential

and psychological emergency: a patient request for a hastening of death. This latter situation would require urgent attention to the patient's experience of illness and, more, an understanding of the significance of the illness within her wider life-story; what has happened to her, how her symptoms are experienced and controlled, and what her concerns, beliefs and expectations are. Put simply, there is a vital and urgent need for a connection or relationship to be established or re-established between the clinician and the individual patient. Negotiating goals of care are still vital, and patient and clinician communication come to the fore as a therapeutic tool.

These complexities of how to best deliver palliative services are not new and it is valuable to examine how issues such as prognosis and patient experiences of illness and its symptoms have been discussed in the past.

Past evidence

Cicely Saunders has been described as the founder of the modern palliative care movement. From the year 1958, new ways of discussing the dying patient were forged and the dying patient was given a voice. Importantly for those involved in the modern palliative care movement, Saunders was one of the few health care workers of the 1950s and 1960s to lobby for death care reform, study pain and analgesia, and give the dying patient a platform and possibly a script from which to speak (Clarke, 1999).

From the 1950s to 1970s, the 'early years' of what was then called terminal or hospice care, professional authoritative opinion loomed large, in contrast to evidence-based medicine. Saunders was a pioneering leader who found evidence of suffering and its relief in literature, theology, poetry, the visual image, and patient story. She was one of the few doctors or nurses in the 1950s who listened to, recorded and wrote about dying patients and their expressions or experience of illness. She recorded patients' accounts with a portable tape recorder and used the transcribed patient narrative to expose the need for death-care reform and to promote the then novel principles of terminal or hospice care (Clarke, 1999). Not only were patient narratives acceptable evidence in these formative years of hospice care, but Cicely Saunders used such evidence of the patient's point of view with telling effect as a vehicle to revolutionize clinical care of the dying. In much of her early writings she uses case studies to illuminate various aspects of caring for dying people.

Communication about prognosis and the patient's heightened awareness of mortality have been, and still are, critical concerns in end-of-life and palliative care which are well reflected in the literature. Cicely Saunders drew attention to these issues through patient narratives which she used in nearly all of her papers and were viewed by her as an essential ingredient in her writings, whether directed to medical or nursing journals. For example, in the *Annals of the Royal College of Surgeons*, Saunders wrote of the perspective of a patient quietly, perhaps obliquely, listening to clinical conversations:

> Patients watch us as we watch them . . . I recall a young woman who, after two months with us, suddenly asked me, "Doctor, where did all this begin?" and then once she was certain of my attention, "What I really wanted to ask you was – is it wrong for me to let my children come up and visit me, now that I am getting so thin?" She well knew both her diagnosis and prognosis for she had learnt them by listening to the round at the end of her bed after a laparotomy some six months earlier, but now she had other questions.
>
> (Saunders, 1967: 165)

This is not simply a narrative that describes and relates a series of events; it is a story that uses plot and emotion for particular effects (see Paley, and Eva this volume). Not only does Saunders want the reader to understand certain types of questions patients have in their minds, she also presents the reader with a view of the patient as a *whole person,* one who listens and is aware of medical consultations at the foot of the bed, and is not simply the passive recipient of medical or nursing care. For example, in 1968 the following was published:

> Very occasionally I am asked a direct question. I remember such a question from Mr Martin whom I knew well and who really wanted a direct answer. When I gave it to him he said, "Was it hard for you to tell me that?" When I said, "Well – yes – it was." He said simply, "Thank you. It is hard to be told, but it is hard to tell too.
>
> (Saunders, 1968: 29)

In this account the reader is brought into a close identification not only with the patient as a whole person with feelings and anxieties, but also with the doctor. Through this confiding account, Saunders, as a doctor, could admit that difficulties arose for her when talking with patients about their impending death. Not merely a neutral, unfeeling professional with expert training and knowledge, the doctor is simultaneously produced and revealed, by Saunders, as both expert and human – as having professional wisdom and specialist knowledge, and feelings and emotions.

Many of Saunders' papers include several different perspectives of evidence which she drew upon to construct a picture of the dying person, his or her suffering and its relief. For example, in a paper from the 1970s entitled *The Nature and Management of Terminal Pain,* Saunders drew on several sources to paint a narrative picture of the patient in chronic pain. The paper is many voiced (Bakhtin, 1981), including first person accounts, third person interpretations by Saunders and some more distant and clinical discussion of the incidence of pain in terminal illness. Also included were transcribed conversational extracts between Saunders and a 'young woman with

metastatic carcinoma of the breast, less than 6 weeks before her death'
(Saunders, 1970a: 25). It reads:

> Dr S: How bad was the pain – that you – were feeling in such need?
>
> Patient: I would say that the pain was so bad that I dreaded anyone touching me and
> when anyone knocked my bed or came near me the first thing I said to them – 'Please
> don't touch me. Please don't move me'.
>
> Dr S: So that was something that really got on top of you – it was really bad?
>
> Patient: Oh yes. I-I-I would say that – it was an obsession in a way because it was all
> round me. I would lie still thinking: 'well, I won't bring it on I will just lie still' and the
> mere fact of everything you did – if you coughed, if you sneezed, if you went to lift
> something, you would find it, you would have it . . .
>
> (Saunders, 1970a: 25)

While the style of writing in the third person can serve to distance the writer
and the reader from whatever is being discussed, in the following cases this
form of narrative construction works to confirm Saunders as an expert. She is
the interpreter for the reader, drawing upon her medical training (perhaps also
her training in social work and nursing) and practical experience to explain the
experiences of dying people to those who are less informed or experienced:

> Another patient said to me, "well, doctor, it began in my back, but now it seems like
> all of me is wrong." And she went on to describe the physical pain, her feelings that
> nobody understood how she felt, that the world was against her, that she could have
> cried for the pills and injections but knew that she should not, that her husband and
> son were having to stay off work to look after her.
>
> (Saunders, 1969: 52–3)

This style of narrative writing has the effect of confirming that the dying patient
is a feeling person; in need, physically and emotionally. Saunders presents
to the reader a view of the patient in pain that transcends a purely physical
understanding of pain. The narrative also sends a strong message to clinicians.
If the patient's pain and suffering were a consequence of being isolated then
sympathetic clinicians could relieve pain, in large part by sensitive understanding of how the patient is feeling and by recognizing the financial impact and
concern for the patient of her husband and son having to stay off work to
care for her. Saunders draws the practitioner into the story when making
a point, both confirming her expertise and but also serving to provide evidence
that her concept of 'total pain' was generated from her interpretations
of patient experiences. In the following passage she reiterates how it is possible
to draw such generalizations from the individual to other patients and the
therapeutic role of the concerned clinician:

> Terminal pain is commonly constant in character and so calls for constant control,
> the titrating of drugs to pain in a particular patient, and its proper timing right

> throughout illness. This demands listening to what the patient has to say in such a way that he finds that you are in alliance with him in his fight against what is going on and that you recognised something of what it all means to him. It is just because of this personal aspect that I am talking from the stories of individual patients. Each one, as it were, illustrates a whole group.
>
> (Saunders, 1970b: 35)

Saunders draws the individual patient, as example, for the reader. She continually uses one patient as the example, to render the notion of the patient in pain, so the clinician can understand any patient more fully. Personal and intimate accounts also served to carry important messages about therapeutic relationships.

Narrative as evidence – potential

What type of evidence, in the climate of evidence-based medicine, can shed light on this therapeutic relationship to enhance or inform professional beliefs, skills, and knowledge? As questions from patients about hastening death are common it is a useful example to continue this discussion. However, patient and clinician stories or narratives are rarely reported in the professional literature concerning how such questions are posed and answered. In fact very little professional literature exists regarding requests for hastening death that can guide practitioners towards best practice.

In the literature that does exist, specific example questions and phrases are offered to give practitioners guidance in how to respond appropriately to patients who request to have their death hastened (Hudson, et al. 2006). For example:

> "Can you tell me about how others have reacted to you being ill like this. . . who would you say understands best what you are going through?"
> . "Could you tell me about the things that you most want to do at this point in your life, the things that you value the most?"
>
> (Hudson, et al. 2006: 708)

The article is produced in an evidence-based framework. Evidence supporting the recommendations was gathered using systematic literature review with expert opinion. The article is a welcome addition to the literature. Yet, in my opinion, I think two things are missing. First, is a focus on human judgement (Hollway, 2001). From the dozens of example phrases, all of which appear reasonable and potentially helpful, individual practitioners using the guidelines will need to add their own personal and professional judgement to the recommendations to choose how to respond to a patient. Such judgement rests on the individual's own personhood, experiences of professional practice and possibly organizational mores, and much more.

Second, is recognition that practitioner and patient are intertwined in the process of making sense of requests for hastening of death. This therapeutic relationship works not in one direction but two (Hollway, 2001). As patient fears are heard and understood in the therapeutic relationship, meanings can be emotionally appreciated, and healing, for the patient, may occur. Likewise, as the professional experience of the practitioner grows, with each patient encounter and each request for hastening of death plus knowledge from systematic reviews, lifelong learning can happen. This learnt astuteness and insight could then be shared with colleagues and larger communities.

Narrative as evidence – complexity

'Will I be alive then?' He asks.

Silence. He sits there looking at me waiting for my answer. Motionless, silent, waiting for me.

I loathe these questions. How many years have I been doing this work? But I hate these questions. Does he sense my unease; inwardly I struggle to think of an answer that won't leave him distraught – to think of an answer that won't turn out untrue. He examines my face since asking his question. Reading my expression, I think. Time seems endless.

What did Dr Marlow say of your illness; did he give you any idea? I say.

I didn't ask him, he always seems so busy and my last appointment up at the hospital was so short. And I reckon that you must see so many people, in situations like mine.' He held his head in his hands and wept, his whole body rocked with his weeping. Then, breathing in deeply he continued, 'I reckon that can't be good.'

I am used to, and contented in fixing, organizing, referring, problem solving, and putting things straight. What can I fix here? Nothing.

He wipes his face, one hand either side, a sweep of his hands and the tears are gone. He sighs deeply again. He doesn't stop crying, he quietly shed occasional tears. He looks to be desperately trying to hold himself together, not to breakdown entirely.

The silence between us grows longer, then, he talks

He would rather be dead now than lumber Mary and Bridget with everything. Somehow I know what is coming, that question.

Can I help him die sooner, he asks?

Silence, my mind races, thinking of the times this has been asked before, this is as difficult now as the first time. Tell me about the girls, I manage to ask. He talks of a father's love and how this is not what he had envisaged, not what he had thought. What did you imagine, I ask. Able and dependable, not disabled and dependent. Just like me, I think to myself. Is this the worst thing right now, I ask, these thoughts of dependency and burdening?

In this story we read of one patient struggling to know what to tell his children of his altered sense of mortality. The strength of the piece is that important information is conveyed in the story: we read that this experienced clinician feels uncomfortable with questions of hastening death; an important message to convey to others – the nature of human professional feelings. No matter the number of years of experience, some interactions and conversations never become straightforward. The description of the patient's emotions is explicit, the personal feelings and expression of them revealed. We read of the clinician reflecting and comparing with the patient.

How can the myriad of potential stories, those made by the writer and all possible readers, help us to understand and grapple with the complexity that is professional palliative care knowledge? This complexity warrants further examination.

Readers of the narrative above will layer their own meaning on the story. For instance, those readers who have received bad news – a forecast of a shortened life, a long wait for biopsy results – to some extent may recall the moments, feelings, and the conversations that happened to them. This imaginative narrative, concocted by the reader in response to what the writer has expressed, will affect the meanings of the narrative above, depending on the reader's experience (Brody, 2003). Readers will always add on to a story's text and may not be aware that they have done so. Clinicians who have been asked to hasten a death will also layer their own experience on the story above. So what of the evidence or truth in the story?

One account of the truth is that the story has face value: this patient felt absolutely dispirited at living with progressive illness; the truth is his expression of his emotions: he felt confused and threatened at the thought of telling his children his fate (Goldie, 2004). This notion of truth, I imagine, will sit comfortably with many palliative care practitioners. Several times every day, a palliative care practitioner believes the perspectives – accepts the points of view and reports of pain and other symptoms – of people she serves, and acts upon them.

Another idea of proof follows. Each reader will have his or her own unique experiences to bear on the story. The idea that all readers of the account above can glean the *same* truth, conjure up the same reaction to his telling of his discussion with the doctor about his diagnosis is highly unlikely. So what does this idea of truth, and the idea of imaginative narrative discussed above, signify to the notion of objectivity? They do not sit comfortably together. This complicates the whole idea of objectivity and the credibility of narrative methods in palliative care.

An elaboration of the story above suggests what objectivity might look like in narrative. For the sake of this elaboration, say that the reader of the story is a young, overworked resident doctor who has just finished a stint on night shift. He might read the story and *diverge in evaluation and emotional response* with the writer's evaluation of events (Goldie, 2004: 162–3). From a 'face value' perspective, the story appears to emphasize the individuality of a response to being sick and aware of mortality. For the young doctor, a quite different, less sympathetic interpretation could be given, that of a man's misplaced question to the doctor. The young doctor sympathizes with the duty of communicating difficult news and remembers past experiences, ill equipped and poorly mentored, with angry patients in the midst of complex needs.

There may be one explanation of objectivity that seems to make sense of this complexity and to its meaning in palliative care. Narrative cannot be devoid of emotion nor can its meanings be the same for different observers/listeners. Indeed, narrative can convey a multiplicity of messages better than other methods; event, emotion, relationship, and the particular rather than the general. The strength of the narrative is that interpretation and judgement happen. Divergence and contestation occurs. Divergence is valuable because it can illuminate the reader's own situation and enable comparisons, scrutiny, and justification of the reader's reactions. As long as one responds more broadly to the narrative in the 'right way' – the response of the reader is the key to objectivity (Goldie, 2004: 164–5). It is about having an appropriate response or opinion to a particular narrative. Appropriate responses are shaped by shared professional beliefs, morals, and expectations regarding human judgements and therapeutic relationships.

Narrative evidence and dialogue

Could narrative evidence be used to improve patient care? Could these appropriate responses be created, nurtured, and used alongside RCT and systematic reviews? For the profession of palliative care this would mean generating a collective story for the discipline that connected and contextualized different professional beliefs, morals, and expectations. Of course, the only way this collective narrative can develop is through a public dialogue about relationships between patient and practitioners – and between practitioners themselves.

Public professional knowledge would be greatly enhanced if narratives were published in which these particular situations and conversations were detailed and described. The discipline would learn how practitioners manage such demanding and critical encounters and it would allow for critical self-reflection and a public dialogue about these essential details: human judgement and therapeutic relationship. It would also enhance the development of a language to discuss such deeply critical issues.

Acknowledgement

Access to Dame Cicely Saunders papers was made possible through the Hospice History Project, Sheffield Palliative Care Studies Group, Department of Palliative Medicine, University of Sheffield, UK.

References

Aoun, S. and Kristjanson, L. (2005) Challenging the framework for evidence in palliative care research. *Palliative Medicine*, **19**(6), 461–65.

Bakhtin, M. (1981) *The Dialogical Imagination: Four Essays*. University of Texas Press Slavic Series, Austin Texas.

Brody, H. (2003) *Stories of Sickness*. Oxford University Press, London.

Clark, D. (1999) 'Total pain', disciplinary power and the body in the work of Cicely Saunders, 1958–1967. *Social Science and Medicine*, **49**, 727–36.

Cochrane, A. (1972) *Effectiveness and Efficiency: Random Reflections on Health Services*. Nuffield Provincial Hospitals Trust.

Devery, K. (2006) The framework for evidence in palliative care: narrative-based evidence. *Palliative Medicine*, **20**(1), 51.

Goldie, P. (2004) Narrative emotion and understanding. In *Narrative Research in Heath and Illness* (eds. B. Hurwitz, T. Greehalgh, and V. Skultans). Blackwell Publishing, Oxford, pp. 156–67.

Gould, S. (1991) 'The Median isn't the Message', in *Bully for Brontosaurus*. Hutchinson Press, London.

Greenhalgh, T. (2004) Meta-narrative mapping: a new approach to the systematic review of complex evidence. In *Narrative Research in Health and Illness* (eds. B. Hurwitz, T. Greehalgh, and V. Skultans). Blackwell Publishing, Oxford, pp. 349–81.

Greenhalgh, T. and Hurwitz, B. (1998) *Narrative based medicine: dialogue and discourse in clinical practice*. British Medical Journal Books, London.

Haynes, R. (2002) What kind of evidence is it that evidence-based medicine advocates want health care providers and consumers to pay attention to? BMC Health Services Research, 2:3, doi:10.1186/1472-6963-2-3. Date viewed 19 February 2008.

Hollway, W. (2001) The psycho-social subject in evidence-based practice. *Journal of Social Work Practice*, **15**(1), 10–22.

Hudson, P., Schofield, P., Kelly, B., Hudson, R., Street, A., O'Connor, M., Kristjanson, L., Ashby, M., and Aranda, S. (2006) Responding to desire to die statements from patients with advanced disease: recommendations for health professionals. *Palliative Medicine*, **20**, 703–10.

Jadad, A. and Rennie, D. (1998) The randomized controlled trial gets a middle-aged checkup. *Journal of the American Medical Association*, **279**, 319–20.

Jennings, A., Davies, A., Higgins, J., and Broadley, K. (2001) Opioids for the palliation of breathlessness in terminal illness. *Cochrane Database of Systematic Reviews* Issue 3. Art. No.: CD002066. doi: 10.1002/14651858.CD002066. Date viewed 16 March 2008.

McAlister, F., van Diepen, S., Padwal, R., Johnson, J., and Majumdar, S. (2007) How evidence-based are the recommendations in evidence-based guidelines? *PLoS Medicine*

Vol. 4, No. 8, e250 doi:10.1371/journal.pmed.0040250. Date viewed 15 March 2008.

National Cancer Institute (2004) Levels of evidence, United States of America. Available at: http://www.cancer.gov/cancertopics/pdq/screening/levels-of-evidence/HealthProfessional/page2 Date viewed 4 March 2008.

National Health and Medical Research Council (2008) Canberra. Available at: http://209.85.141.104/search?q=cache:P7iiP9VBNucJ:www.nhmrc.gov.au/consult/add_levels_grades_dev_guidelines2.htm±levels±of±evidence±site:nhmrc.gov.auandhl=enandct=clnkandcd=2andgl=au Date viewed 26 June 2008.

Phillips, B., Ball, C., Sackett, D., Badenoch, D., Straus, S., Haynes, B., and Dawes, M. (2001) Oxford centre for evidence-based medicine levels of evidence, Centre for evidence-based medicine, Oxford, United Kingdom, www.cebm.net/index.aspx?o=1047 Date viewed 26 June 2008.

Rothwell, P., (2005) External validity of randomised controlled trials: "To whom do the results of this trial apply?" *Lancet*, **365**, 82–93.

Sackett, D. and Roseberg, W. (1995) The need for evidence based medicine. *Journal of the Royal Society of Medicine.* Nov; **88**(11), 620–24.

Sackett, D., Rosenberg, W., Gray, J., Haynes, R., and Richardson, W. (1996) *Evidence-based Medicine: What it is and What it isn't* (Editorial), *British Medical Journal*, **312**(7023), 71–72.

Saunders, C. (1967) The care of the terminal stages of cancer. *Annals of the Royal College of Surgeons.* **41** supplement, 162–69.

Saunders, C. (1968) The last stages of life. *Recover*, Summer, 26–29.

Saunders, C. (1969) The moment of truth: care of the dying person. In *Death and Dying: Current Issues In The Treatment Of The Dying Person* (ed. L. Pearson). The Press of Case Western Reserve, Cleveland, Ohio, pp. 49–78.

Saunders, C. (1970a) The nature and management of terminal pain. In *Matters of Life and Death* (ed. E. Shotter). Darton, Longman and Todd, London, pp.15–26.

Saunders, C. (1970b) An individual approach to the relief of pain. In *People and Cancer.* The British Cancer Council, London, pp.34–8.

Seale, C. (1998) *Constructing Death*, Cambridge University Press. Cambridge.

Timmermans, S. and Berg, M. (2003), *The Challenge of Evidence based Medicine and Standardisation in Health Care.* Temple University Press, Philadelphia.

Chapter 5

Therapeutic writing: 'writing is a way of saying things I can't say'

Gillie Bolton

The exploratory study discussed in this chapter began a unique process of qualitative enquiry into therapeutic creative writing and its value to patients in palliative care and oncology settings. The study sought to illuminate patients' experiences of personal creative writing and the existential criteria they used to describe their writing experiences.

My personal experience of creative writing with patients is that it can be a powerful therapeutic tool. Writing can help very sick people understand themselves better, think through issues, memories, feelings, and thoughts; accommodate to what is happening to them better; and communicate more effectively with significant others. It also offers the focused satisfaction of involvement in an artistic process. This involvement can enable patients to tolerate or modulate anxiety, pain, and fear. It can also redirect individuals towards an appreciation of life, and give them a sense of achievement and authority in a valued sphere. Such writers are not, however, concerned to create artistic products; the focus of the work is on the process of doing it.

The power of creative writing for personal development is well documented (Hunt and Sampson, 2006; Progoff, 1975), and has long been attested to by writers (Middlebrook, 1992; Woolf, 1977, 1978, 1980). Expressive writing on subjects of significance to the writer has been found to improve health outcomes significantly (McGuire, et al. 2005), and to alleviate distress (Smyth, 1998). Other research (Bolton, 1999; Bolton, et al. 2000; Smyth, et al. 1999; Lepore and Smyth, 2002; and see below) indicates that deeply expressive and explorative writing can ease symptoms because the psychological and the physical are so closely linked, an effect related to the well-known placebo phenomenon.

All the patients involved in the study discussed here, indicated that they found therapeutic writing beneficial, saying, for example that 'it made it less traumatic than it might have been otherwise'. Data analysis showed that writing facilitated three main processes: first, a reflection upon internal issues (e.g. what patients thought, felt, remembered) and external ones (e.g. relation-ships, events, nature); second, communication not only with the self, but also with significant others such as medical and health care staff and relatives; and third, responses to the creative process, such as a sense of pride or achievement – everyone feels better when they've made something. The staff member 'essays' offered insight into a range of benefits to patients as well as the intrinsic value of staff writing groups.

Therapeutic creative writing: principles and practice

Therapeutic writing can help individuals to understand themselves and their situations better, and deal with depression, distress, anxiety, fear of disease, treatment, and the changes necessitated by illness and dying. The emphasis is on processes to create material of satisfaction and interest to the writer, and possibly a few close others. Not only patient-participative (Farrell and Gilbert, 1996), it is also patient-directed. Patients or clients are offered guidance and inspiration by a clinician or creative writer, and support in choosing subject and form. Each writer works according to his/her personal interests, concerns, wants, and needs. Authority and control of each piece of writing always resides with the writer, to re-read and re-work, share with appropriate others or not, store unread, or possibly destroy.

There are five foundational principles which patients embrace when writing therapeutically. These are: (i) trust in the processes of writing which taps into the wise strong part of oneself; (ii) self-respect for oneself as a writer, however brief it may be; (iii) responsibility to take authority over the products of writing and the learning; (iv) generosity to the self in giving time to enjoy and learn from these pursuits; (v) positive regard for the family, friends, and professionals who are written about and reflected upon.

Individuals can write in their own time and space, with the support and guidance of appropriate staff (health care, writer, or researcher). They then choose with whom to share their writing and experiences – previous studies have shown much writing is shared with family or friends, and that not all is shared with staff (Bolton, 1999; Hannay and Bolton, 2000).

Previous research

Research has shown that personally disclosive writing, undertaken under trial conditions with healthy individuals is associated with the mood and quality of life benefits (Van Zuuren, et al. 1999), and with patients is associated with such factors as an increase in immune function (Lepore and Smyth, 2002). An editorial concerning Smyth et al.'s (1999) research stated that 'Were the authors to have provided similar outcome evidence about a new drug, it likely would be in widespread use within a short time. Why? We would think we understood the "mechanism" (whether we did or not) and there would be a mediating industry to promote its use' (Spiegel, 1999). Such studies of writing interventions have typically asked subjects to write about traumatic or stressful experiences in a research, rather than therapeutic setting (Broderick, et al. 2005; Smyth, et al. 1999), an approach not considered appropriate, nor useful to palliative or oncology patients.

Our research

Our study differed in nature and focus from previous research in non-palliative care settings. These previous studies have demonstrated that disclosure through set expressive writing tasks (usually in a laboratory setting) seems to have measurable effects at a physiological level, as well as demonstrable mental and physical health outcomes (Pennebaker and Chung, 2007). The methods used in our study involved encouragement to write, and suggestions for writing topics rather than set tasks. Each patient was offered support and advice – individually or in small groups – about the writing they might undertake. We however took the findings of wider studies (Broderick, et al. 2005; Lepore and Smyth, 2002; Petrie, et al. 1998; Smyth, 1999; Van Zuuren, et al. 1999) to be indicative: some of the value of writing in the palliative care setting may emanate from its disclosive potential.

Our study offered an open-ended, supported opportunity for patients to write in whatever way, and about whatever subject appropriate to them; disclosure was not central. This approach to therapeutic writing has a clear background in, and links to, artistic creative writing methods. Works of artistic merit such as poetry can be created by this kind of process; although not its focus: 'Poems . . . profoundly alter the man or woman who wrote them' (Abse, 1998: 362); 'Every poem breaks a silence that had to be overcome' (Rich, 1995: 84).

Previous qualitative research with depressed primary care patients (Hannay and Bolton, 2000), hospice patients (Bolton, 1999), and counselling clients (Wright, 2003, 2005a&b, 2006) show similar results to our study. Research with women with breast cancer indicated positive effects (Stanton, et al. 2002). Considerable research has been undertaken with a wide range of patient and subject groups including the positive effect of writing on the success of young romantic relationships (Slatcher and Pennebaker (2006) have undertaken an overview of current research). Poetry writing is used in cancer and chronic illness (Elfick and Head, 2004; Miller, 2001; Mirriam-Goldberg, 2004;

Schneider, 2003), and haiku writing in palliative care in Japan (Tamba, 2004). Schwartz and David (2002) tell us:

> Clinicians have noted that [cancer] patients [during their last year of life] do not discuss their dying unless they are given a context in which to do so (Kubler Ross, 1969), and that when patients are given opportunities to shift their focus to inner life concerns – existential and relational concerns – then a sense of preparedness for coping with mortality may enhance emotional well-being during this poignant period (Bynock, 1997; Groopman, 1997). When cancer patients focus on the medical at the exclusion of other facets of their lives, we believe that they miss critical opportunities to address the emotional and existential issues that would lead to intimacy with loved ones and closure. These issues are critical to improving quality of life at the end of life and in fact have recently been documented as being core attributes to a "good death" experience for 81–90% of patients (Steinhauser, et al. 2000). In the spirit of facilitating this process, we have developed a written expression intervention that seeks to provide patients with a vehicle for processing the emotional and existential issues that arise in the face of the later stages of a terminal illness.
>
> (Schwartz and David, 2002: 258)

Although the intervention described here was appropriately facilitative, in-depth and creative, and was clearly valuable, this was a quantitative study on such a tiny sample (12 patients) that the outcomes are not useful. Qualitative data, such as personal meaning, were not obtained.

The writers in the study, and the circumstances of their writing

The study involved 13 teenage cancer patients and 11 community palliative care cancer patients (40 years and older) who undertook different sorts of writing in a range of settings. They wrote stories (fictional and semi-fictional), including poetry, personal journal entries, autobiographical accounts, descriptions of their homes, wards, and experiences of cancer and treatment. I worked with them in workshop settings (up to 8 teenage cancer patients in the Unit day-room); individually at the bedside, in their homes (community patients), and in the Unit dayroom. Much of the writing was undertaken alone and read to me later. Involvement in the project was entirely optional. Authority and control of each piece of writing resided with each writer, who gave signed consent to their involvement in the study, and to publication of their writings and interview transcripts. Those who undertook three pieces of writing were invited to write an evaluative 'essay' 'what this writing has meant to me', and be interviewed by a voluntary experienced research interviewer; interviews were transcribed.

My content interpretation and analysis of patient essays, writing and interview transcripts indicated significant elements concerning the personal value or impact of the writing processes. I then studied these alongside my field-notes for themes and narrative lines which explicitly or implicitly seemed to offer insight into the therapeutic writing process: the way it had been used by the patient, and its possible functions and effects. The analytic and interpretative focus was consistently the personal and developmental: artistic value was frequently present, but was not the focus of enquiry. Following an initial sensitisation process, the Project Steering Group discussed data analysis in order to bring wider perspectives.

Two staff writing groups, run in each setting, offered staff experiential knowledge and understanding of the processes. One staff member in each setting was invited to write an 'essay', 'What this writing meant to my patients and colleagues', to give professional background in the report.

The research data offer insight into the value of writing to patients: benefits, disadvantages and harms associated with therapeutic writing in these settings. The enquiry process was based on narrative approaches (Hillman, 1986, 1997). Narrative analysis has been seen as an 'empowering' social science methodology, paying attention to the subjects' expression of their own viewpoints and evaluative standards. It focuses upon how the past shapes perceptions of the present, how the present influences the way past is seen, and how both shape orientation to the future (McAdams, 1993; Riesman, 1993). All material was scrutinized for either expressed or implicit value and function. Elements and interpretations drawn from the four forms of data by me, were in turn examined and discussed by the research steering group.

Research steering and management groups met regularly. They supported, advised, and oversaw the project. They included two medical (clinical) academics with experience of Medical Humanities and the healing arts, an experienced academic medical qualitative researcher, a professor of Higher Education, a literature officer from the Arts Council England, and myself.

Extracts from patient writings, interview transcripts, patient and staff *essays*, and researcher's field-notes illuminate the following examination of cancer patients' writing and how they reported its personal meaning.

Patients' experience of writing

A particular quality of explorative and expressive writing is that it is private until the writer chooses to share it: 'not really for anyone else other than yourself', as one patient put it. Personal writing is tentative: 'If it's written only for the self, then it can be un-said', said in different ways, or it can be deleted and the opposite tried instead. Its impermanence is an essential element: this is process work, not writing for a literary product, though the artifact in progress can be extremely important to the writer.

An expression of the otherwise inexpressible seems to be enabled. The quietness of writing, and there being no immediate listener unlike in oral narratives, seems be conducive. 'Writing is a way of saying things I can't say. I do it when I'm on my own, and as a way of coping with being down. I know I mustn't give in to being down and give in to the cancer and writing helps.'

The content is generally spontaneous and written 'in a fairly haphazard, unstructured kind of way'. 'I write without pre-censoring what I will say', with 'recklessness, in a moment of madness'.

These very sick or terminally ill people said that they had a 'mass of jumbled thoughts and feelings'. Writing in this way can help to 'put it in some sort of order'. It gets these 'things which swirl around my head' 'outside' where 'it will be easier to deal with', 'instead of just keeping them like bottled up'.

Many people felt the process 'unburdened' them; 'what's within me is externalised, is deposited outside myself'; 'words on a page are one of the dustbin men'. All these expressions give a sense of service rendered by the writing: dustbin men remove unwanted waste; an un-carryable load is taken away. These and other patients filled in more about how writing then deals with this 'burden' or 'dustbin material': one patient said it 'took me some way towards purging it and integrating it into my life'. 'Purging' and 'integrating it into my life' may appear to be contradictory, but I think this writer meant similar to those who said: 'once it's outside its easier to deal with'. And 'I do find it easier to talk about it now'. It seems that writing can purge (unburden, release from being bottled, empty from the dustbin) this personal material from an inaccessible internal lodging, to where it can be dealt with, talked about and reflected upon, sometimes being repositioned 'in some sort of order'. These writers did not read each other's *essays* or interview transcripts on how they felt about the writing, so it's interesting so many expressed themselves in such similar metaphors. This might relate to the psychologist Bruner's theory of 'cannonical narratives'(1990) which he saw as relating to wider social expectations.

Such writing was not easy: thoughts, feelings, and memories were not lightly given to the 'dustbin men': 'the writing process allowed me to discover the things that were still problems and unresolved issues in my mind . . . [it] brought a lot of simmering and difficult emotions to the surface.' Yet these writers felt that it was worth it, the same person finishing his *essay* with 'so it's been a good experience for me', and another 'writing is a safe vehicle for recklessness'. Aristotle speaks of watching a poetic tragedy on the stage 'producing through the pity and fear caused, a catharsis of those emotions' (Aristotle, trans. 1996). One of the writers spoke of their writing as cathartic, and two others as purgative (the literal translation of cathartic). The cathartic stage of experiencing these extremely painful feelings, and the ensuing stages of reflecting upon them were all disturbing and painful, highlighting the need for emotional support.

A very young teenage cancer patient, an asylum seeker who had lost all her family except her sister, started writing about her home and family memories. She dissolved in tears, and was prevented from continuing due to a medical intervention. On a subsequent occasion her eyes followed me round the ward until I hesitatingly went to her to ask if she'd like to try again. Her eyes brightened. Despite little English and desperate tears, she started again with the same words and wrote her heartrending piece. It begins: 'In my house in Angola we had a lot of beautiful flowers because my mum said the flowers bring peace at home, and she liked that so much.' Her *essay* about the writing later was merely: 'I like doing it a lot. I like to remember. I like to think about it.'

A further common theme was how the creative process was related to pride and enhanced self-respect and confidence: 'I'm proud and stimulated by some of the things I've written'; 'It's something I have done myself. No-one can correct me. It's mine. It doesn't matter if it's right or wrong.'

A staff member who contributed to the qualitative data wrote:

> As for the work with patients I thought it was fantastic on so many levels. Having someone new, who was so confident in what they were doing, became a feature of the week that many patients looked forward to. The writing sessions were a welcome addition to the routine of activities and were offered in a very approachable way that many patients felt able to try. In at least one instance a patient had not been able to verbalise his feelings but found he could express them in writing and went on to use art as well. It was deeply personal and private for him and I believe he was much more at peace for it. For others it highlighted issues that they perhaps were not aware were as important as they were i.e. when describing characters in a story one patient always seemed to concentrate on the girl's hair. The patient had thought she herself was fine about her own hair loss and the stories raised it as an issue for her that she was then able to talk about and accept better. The writing definitely affected other activities such as the patient group; patients who had written together talked much more easily together than they had previously.
>
> The great thing about the writing is that the writer is in control every step of the way. It was presented in a non-threatening and non-pushy way, which helped everyone to feel safe.
>
> I found the whole experience enriching and enormously positive. The writing is a hugely powerful tool, which enables people to get in touch with themselves at a level that is much deeper than many were expecting.

Web logging (Blogging)

A palliative care cancer patient emailed me after I'd visited:

> A few ideas came into my head the moment you walked out the door last week. I finished up writing something. It just all came out as one fat lump. First draft. Finished. I put it straight onto my website.

TERMINAL. 11/3/04.
Have I been abandoned,
Or in the scheme of things, just set free,
Like cherry tree blossom on the air,
Or a leaf dropped upon
The turbulent surface of a stream.

Its not that my doctors don't care.
What more can they do.

I could turn, stretch out my arms
And say "don't leave me on my own,
I'm ill and feel secure with you there".

But I'm the one going to die.
The one bringing tears to the eyes of children.

So in an effort to understand
Why we finish up alone,
I must rationalise my fears
And become strong.

Blogs go out to an audience of anyone, as this writer made clear on his website: 'After starting to tell you about the problems of my early teens, I feel a great relief. Some of the pressure, the need to spill more of the beans has gone, but there is more that needs to be said. Those events had a negative effect on me and the way I've lived my life.' By 'tell' he means post on the web. 'You' is his audience out there – strangers as well as known people such as family, friends, and me. The web might be public, but it is also impermanent. Such personal writing is open to being rewritten, rethought. This plastic quality is an essential therapeutic element: 'there's always an option to un-write'.

Poetry

The writing above, which 'just all came out as one fat lump. 'First draft. Finished' came out in poetic form. It often does. '*First draft. Finished*' poetry seems to be conducive to people exploring vital existential thoughts, feelings, and experiences. Quick and succinct, poetry does not need to have the bulky prose structure of sentences, paragraphs and reaching the right-hand page margin; and it can leap from one idea or image to another. This speed of first draft composition, which can enable a grasping of psychologically elusive but vital images, thoughts, feelings, experiences, is not specific to therapeutic writers. Here Seamus Heaney writes of the process of another great poet:

> Czeslaw Milosz's frequent claim that his poems were dictated by a daimon, that he was merely a 'secretary'. Which was another way of saying that he had learned to write fast, to allow the associative jumps to be taken at a hurdler's pace.
>
> (Heaney, 2004: 6)

For some, poetry is not always the right medium for the expression of strong experiences such as bereavement. Poet Mark Doty explains why he wrote *Heaven's Coast* (Doty, 1996) in prose. 'Poetry was too tight, too contained for the amount of emotion I had to express when Wally died. I wallowed in sentences, they were deeply satisfying' (Personal Communication).

Poetry, furthermore, uses image as a medium of expression and mode of exploration (Modell, 1997). Are cherry blossom or autumn leaves abandoned when they fall, or are they a free beautiful gift from nature? 'Like cherry tree blossom on the air, / Or a leaf dropped upon / The turbulent surface of a stream.' If these lines were omitted, the poem would lose significance and be less memorable beginning only with 'Have I been abandoned, / Or in the scheme of things, just set free'. The single word *turbulent* is important; put in the right place it affects the whole poem.

The poem below by a 14-year-old cancer patient is full of imagery, with a story just beginning at the end. Note how it moves from the outside cold and dreary images to the hopeful joyful inside. Another patient similarly found writing helped him 'consider the value and quality of whatever you're doing now':

Darkness, cold weather, damp and dreary
Sleet and rain
Cold toes and feet
Brown and green trees in thick deep and white snow
Owls deer and foxes

Christmas carols and bells
The colour of tinsel
The smell and taste of Christmas cooking
Drinks of all sorts

Tommy wears a red Christmas hat
with a white bobble on the end
a shirt, a jumper, brown trousers and trainers
His job is to set up the Christmas tree
Putting up the actual tree, the lights
Putting presents under the tree.

Story

Writing seems to enable the creation and telling of valuable stories, to the self and possibly also to others. Stories are our human filing system: we don't store data as in a computer, we story it. Once storied, complex events can take on an appearance of greater coherence and comprehensibility.

Everyone has some sort of story of their life. They feel they know who they are, where they came from, and have some account of where they think they are going. Illness, terminal diagnosis, or bereavement can inevitably make this previously workable story no longer functional or even broken (Frank, 1995); 'I might never see my grandchildren', for example. Previous hopes and fears, plans and aspirations can become irrelevant. Considering the story of their life, in a form which includes the illness, bereavement or possibility of death or disablement, can enable people to make greater sense of their new lives (Bolton, 2005; Charon, 2001; Charon and Montello, 2002).

Fiction or autobiography

Many patients wrote about events in their lives, seeking to make some sort of sense in the writing. C wrote about the death of his mother, comparing it with his own experience of cancer, and trying to work out the significance of her dying of the same disease while he was so very ill himself. Here is an extract from my field-notes:

> C said he used the writing to help him to regain a hold on reality. He felt he'd lost the plot in his life, was identifying too closely and muddlingly with other people he knew with cancer. He found it very useful when I suggested that the illness has made him lose the plot of his life, by disrupting it so thoroughly. I suggested he's writing to 'heal his story' (Brody, 2003; Frank, 1995). He found this metaphor very useful.

Some write fiction. Master S only wrote the one poem above for this research. All the rest of his writing was fiction. Here is the final section of a story about a 5-year-old protagonist:

> The other children that he had made friends with on the ward were very friendly and talkative. They knew each other for about a year now, and they were ready to do anything for each other because they had gone through so much together, experienced so many pains together.
>
> The next day the organisers introduced a singer who brings the children some presents. He sings pop music, and he's been on Top of the Pops. His songs have been number 1. He also does many charity events, concerts, and he loves children. With him he brings copies of his albums with diskmans – one for everyone. And autographed pictures, and photographs and things like that. All the children are really excited when he sings live for them.
>
> He has heard about Ben's sleeping problem and he tells him that everything will be ok. He tells him to listen to his music and that'll help him sleep. He tells him to just think of ideas at night for stories – could be anything – adventure, fantasy, horror – like the story they heard read at night. And he tells him that the ones he wants to remember maybe he can write them in his diary or something the next day. He suggests Ben might write a diary about what's been happening.
>
> Ben is amazed at what the superstar is telling him and he is surprised at how much the guy knows about him and his life. In the common-room after hearing the story all the children and the nurses say goodnight to each other with hugs and kisses and retire to their beds. As Ben wasn't sleepy he reflected back on the words of the superstar. And he decided to write a diary. First he wrote about his

parents and his family being there for him all the time. He dedicated a number of pages to his kittens for being there no matter what happened, even when he was in trouble.

He wrote about all of his friends, his superstar, all that had happened on the first day. He wrote about the nurses taking care of him well, activities taking place, and what he planned to do ahead. He writes a couple of lines about the surroundings and the countryside. He thinks he can cope with it now, and people have comforted him and told him of techniques he can use.

He came back to the present and dreaded the moments when his parents would leave him. He lifted up his diskman, put the headphones in his ears and slowly closed his eyes.

I quote from my research field-notes:

Master S, an extremely polite, serious, charming 14 year old, whose school work was nearly always scientific. Yet this long story was written on several occasions. His little protagonist is very young, yet he bravely tackles his fear and isolation in the story situation (one similar to the writer's cancer ward). And he is helped by an authority figure – a pop star. He used his little character's struggles and life successes to say things to himself. A 5 year old can be frightened and accept such help. Master S can accept it on the 5 year old character's behalf.

Master S was always very definite about his stories. I made an error once in typing because I couldn't read the writing. He very politely told me he must have said it wrong before, but what he *meant* was. . . . He then repeated exactly what he'd written the week before. Yet despite this clarity and certainty, he often used the provisional tense – maybe the character did certain things. Does he live his life in maybe? The pop star is the wise person who knows Ben inside, and can offer wise advice. The pop star knowing about Ben's sleeping problem came quite out of the blue; the story shifted emphasis and importance from then.

This young fiction writer was using his story to hear the strong wise authority figure in his own head: the pop star is his own wise strong self.

Conclusion

These cancer and palliative patients found that therapeutic creative writing helped them explore and express intensely personal thoughts feelings and experiences, reflect upon relationships, events, and the natural world, communicate painful or personally vital elements with significant others, and gain a sense of pride and achievement in creation. Engaging in writing processes similar to the initial stages of literary writing, as well as talking about their writing, provided important reflection at a significant stage of their lives. 'I, being poor, have only my dreams;/I have spread my dreams under your feet' (Yeats, 1899). Our sleeping dreams, and waking ones expressed in writing, are our riches. To find them spread openly under our feet, we only need basic literacy, pen, and paper.

Acknowledgements

Deep thanks are due to the patients who so generously gave their time and fragile energy. To the staff who were so supportive. To University College Hospital London Myerstein Institute of Oncology and Teenage Cancer Trust Unit, Camden Palliative Care Unit, King's College London English Department, and Arts Council England for enabling this study into a vital un-researched area. Finally to the members of the Research Steering Group. A version of this chapter was first published in *Journal of Medical Ethics: Medical Humanities*, vol. 34 no. 1, June 2008.

References

Abse, D. (1998) More than a green placebo. *The Lancet*, **351**(9099), 362–64.

Aristotle (trans. 1996) *Poetics* (trans. Heath, M.) Penguin, London, p. 10 [49b27].

Bolton, G., Gelipter, D., and Nelson, P. (2000) Keep taking the words: therapeutic writing in primary care. *British Journal of General Practice*, **50**(450), 80–81.

Bolton, G. (1999) *The Therapeutic Potential of Creative Writing: Writing Myself*. Jessica Kingsley Publishers, London.

Bolton, G. (2005) *Reflective Practice Writing and Professional Development*. Sage Publications, London.

Broderick, J. E., Doerte, U., Junghaenel, M. A., and Schwartz, J. E. (2005) Written emotional expression produces health benefits in fibromyalgia patients. *Psychosomatic Medicine*, **67**, 326–34.

Brody, H. (2003) *Stories of Sickness* (2nd edn), Oxford University Press, Oxford.

Bruner, J. (1990) *Acts of Meaning*. Cambridge, Harvard University Press, Massachusetts.

Bynock, I. (1997) *Dying Well: The Prospect for Growth at the End of Life*, Riverhead Books, New York.

Charon, R. and Montello, M. (2002) *Stories Matter: The Role of Narrative in Medical Ethics*. Routledge, New York.

Charon, R. (2001) Narrative medicine: form function and ethics. *Annals of Internal Medicine*, **134**(1), 83–87.

Doty, M. (1996) *Heaven's Coast: A Memoir*. Harpercollins, New York.

Elfick, H. and Head, D. (2004) *Attending to the Fact: Staying with Dying*. Jessica Kingsley Publishers, London.

Farrell, C. and Gilbert, C. (1996) *Health Care Partnerships*. Kings Fund, London.

Frank, A. (1995) *The Wounded Storyteller: Body, Illness and Ethics*. University of Chicago Press, Chicago.

Groopman, J. (1997) *The Measure of Our Days: New Beginnings at Life's End*. Viking, New York.

Hannay, D. and Bolton, G. (2000) Therapeutic writing in primary care: a feasibility study. *Primary Care Psychiatry*, **5**, 157–60.

Heaney, S. (2004) In gratitude for the gifts. *Guardian Review*. 11 September 2004, pp. 4–6.

Hillman, J. (1986) *Healing Fictions*. Spring Publications, Putnam CT.

Hillman, J. (1997) *Archetypal Psychology*. Spring Publications, Putnam CT.

Hunt, C. and Sampson, F. (2006) *Writing Self and Reflexivity*. Palgrave Macmillan, Basingstoke Hampshire.

Kubler Ross, E. (1969) *On Death and Dying*. Macmillan, New York.

Lepore, S. and Smyth, J. M. (eds) (2002) *The Writing Cure*. American Psychological Association, Washington DC.

McAdams, D. P. (1993) *The Stories We Live By: Personal Myths and the Making of the Self*. William C. Morrow and Co, New York.

McGuire, K. M. B., Greenberg, M. A., and Gevirtz, R. (2005) Autonomic effects of expressive writing in individuals with elevated blood pressure. *Journal of Health Psychology*, **10**, 197–207.

Middlebrook, D. W. (1992) *Anne Sexton: A Biography*. Virago, London.

Miller, K. (2001) *The Cancer Poetry Project*. Fairview Press, Minneapolis.

Mirriam-Goldberg, C. (2004) Cancer and chronic illness: a brief report. *Journal of Poetry Therapy*, **17**(2), 101–07.

Modell, A. H. (1997) Reflections on metaphor and affects. *Annals of Psychoanalysis*, **25**, 219–33.

Pennebaker J. W. and Chung, C. K. (2007) Expressive writing, emotional upheavals, and health. In *Handbook of Health Psychology* (eds. H. Friedman and R. Silver). Oxford University Press, New York.

Pennebaker, J. W. and Chung, C. K. (2007) Expressive writing, emotional upheavals, and health. In *Handbook of Health Psychology* (eds. H. Friedman and R. Silver). Oxford University Press, New York, pp. 263–84.

Petrie, K. J, Booth, R. J., and Pennebaker J. W (1998) The immunological effects of thought suppression. *Journal of Personality and Social Psychology*, **75**(5), 1264–72.

Progoff, I. (1975) *At a Journal Workshop*. Dialogue House Library, New York.

Rich, A. (1995) *What is Found There: Notebooks on Poetry and Politics*. Virago, London, p. 84.

Riesman, C. K. (1993) *Narrative Analysis*. Sage Publications, London.

Sartre, J. P. (1938 [1963]) Penguin, Middlesex, *Nausea*.

Schneider, M. (2003) *Writing my Way through Cancer*. Jessica Kingsley, London.

Schwartz, C. E. and David, E. (2002) To everything there is a season: a written expression intervention for closure at the end of life. In *The Writing Cure* (eds. S. Lepore and J.M. Smyth). American Psychological Association, Washington DC, pp. 257–78.

Slatcher, R. B., and Pennebaker, J. W. (2006) How do I love thee? Let me count the words: The social effects of expressive writing. *Psychological Science*, **17**(8), 685–95.

Smyth, J. M., Stone, A., Hurewitz, A., and Kaell, A. (1999) Effects of writing about stressful experiences on symptom reduction in patients with asthma or rheumatoid arthritis. *Journal of the American Medical Association*, **281**(14), 1304–09.

Smyth, J. M. (1998) Written emotional expression: Effect sizes, outcome types, and moderating variables. *Journal of Consulting and Clinical Psychology*, **66**, 174–84.

Spiegel, D. (1999) Editorial: Healing words: emotional expression and disease outcome. *Journal of the American Medical Association*, **281**(14), 1328–29.

Stanton, A. L., Danoff-Burg S., Sworowski, L. A, Collins, C. A., Branstetter, A. D., Rodrigues-Hanley, A., Kirk, S. B., and Austenfeld, J. L. (2002) Randomised controlled trial of written emotional expression and benefit finding in breast cancer patients. *Journal of Clinical Oncology*, **20**(20), 4160–68.

Steinhauser, K. E., Kristakis, N. A., Clipp, E. C., McNeilly McIntyre. L., and Tulsky, J. A. (2000) Factors considered important at the end of life by patients, family, physicians and other careproviders. *Journal of the American Medical Association*, **284**, 2476–82.

Tamba, K. (2004) The use of personalised poems in palliative care: on Japanese health professional's experience. *International Journal of Palliative Nursing*, **10**(11), 534–36.

Woolf, V. (1977, 1978, 1980) *The Diary of Virginia Woolf*. Vols 1, 2 and 3. Hogarth Press, London.

Wright, J. K. (2003) Five Women talk about work-related brief therapy and therapeutic writing. *Counselling and Psychotherapy Research*, **3**, 204–09.

Wright, J. K. (2005a) Writing on prescription? Using writing in brief therapy. *Healthcare Counselling and Psychotherapy Journal*. October Issue, 28–30.

Wright, J. K. (2005b) Writing therapy in brief workplace counselling, *Counselling and Psychotherapy Research*, **5**, 111–19.

Wright, J. K. (2006) A practice of writing. *British Journal of Psychotherapy Integration*, Special Issue on Narrative, **2**(2), 39–48.

Yeats, W. B. (1974 [1899]) He wishes for the embroidered cloths of heaven. In *Selected Poetry*. Macmillan, London, p. 35.

Van Zuuren, F. J., Schoutrop, M. J. A., Lange, A., Louis, C. M., and Slegers, J. E. M. (1999) Effective and ineffective ways of writing about traumatic experiences: a qualitative study. *Psychotherapy Research*, **9**(3), 363–80.

Section 2

Services and care

Chapter 6

Narrative, story, and service evaluation – patients' stories and their consequences

Gail Eva

The ideas of 'narrative' and 'story' represent a rich resource in health care, both in the provision of clinical care (e.g. Barnard et al. 2000; Devery, 2006; Greenhalgh and Hurwitz, 1998; Maddocks, 2003; Quill, 1996) and in research (Frank, 2000; Hurwitz et al. 2002). However, the focus of much of this valuable work is on the contribution of narrative to an understanding of the individual and their experience of health and illness. This chapter, by contrast, will explore the use of narrative – in the specific form of stories – in understanding and evaluating the delivery of a health care service. I will suggest an approach which draws on techniques used in literary criticism to demonstrate the way in which the textual features of a story can account for its particular effects. I will use, as an example, a study of the provision of rehabilitation to patients with metastatic spinal cord compression to show how the interaction between patients' stories and health care professionals' responses contributed significantly to a shortage of meaningful help with managing disability. I will begin with a brief account of the problem observed, and follow this with a discussion of speech act theory, before, finally, applying this to the stories told by two specific patients. *The names of the patients have been changed, and identifying details anonymized.*

Accounting for an unintended outcome

It is well known that metastatic spinal cord compression is a cause of significant disability (Cowap et al. 2000; Kirshblum et al. 2001; McKinley et al. 1999), and there is evidence that rehabilitation interventions can assist patients with this condition in maximizing their independence and contributing to patients' well-being (Catz et al. 2004; Eriks et al. 2004; Guo et al. 2003; Tang et al. 2007).

Consequently, in most centres where patients with spinal cord compression are treated, some provision will be made for rehabilitation. This was certainly the case at one regional cancer centre in the United Kingdom, where services were set up to provide nursing, occupational therapy, physiotherapy, and social work both on the in-patient units and in the community. However, in a study of the extent to which patients were receiving these services, it was found that very few patients were, in fact, being provided with any meaningful rehabilitation (the details of this research have been reported elsewhere: Eva, 2006, 2007).

The obvious question that arises is: why? If the benefits of a particular intervention are accepted, and services are in place to provide it, why are patients not receiving it? Here are a few candidate answers: staffing levels could be inadequate, staff might not have sufficient training in cancer rehabilitation, facilities for rehabilitation might be less than ideal, or there could be poor coordination between the various agencies providing rehabilitation. The problem with these answers is that they are highly unspecific. They are 'off the peg' explanations, readily available, convenient, and capable of being wheeled out to cover any eventuality. In the particular situation under scrutiny here, one could make a case for all of these factors being at least partially present; but, one could also give an equally accurate account of a service which was well-structured and well-coordinated, with senior, experienced rehabilitation staff in post, an effective weekly multidisciplinary team meeting, and where staff – including senior doctors and ward management – valued rehabilitation and were committed to its provision.

More staff, more training, more time would not obviously produce better outcomes. However, we are still left with the problem of accounting for a situation where, despite the life-changing consequences of disability for this group of patients, despite the best intentions of the health care staff concerned, and despite the fact that the necessary arrangements are in place, very few patients with spinal cord compression were receiving support in adjusting to life with a disability. A more fruitful line of enquiry than identifying barriers or deficiencies is to draw on Pawson and Tilley's (1997) 'context-mechanism-outcome' (CMO) model to understand the ways in which particular configurations of attitudinal, institutional, and social processes produce a range of outcomes in different contexts. According to Pawson and Tilley's account, outcomes result from the interactions between stakeholders, interventions, and environments. The potentially desirable outcome – in this case, people with spinal cord compression being able to fulfil their desired roles in their families or communities – will be dependent on the interaction of a number of variables: prognosis, level of disability, coping mechanisms, family support, community support, and many more. Rather than listing factors, we should instead examine how they link together – like ropes, pulleys, and cog wheels, to use Elster's (1989) metaphor – in a certain structure. The analysis of mechanisms does not involve suggesting that there is not enough of one or more resources; it involves pointing out how each component connects up with others to produce a particular result.

In the evaluation of this rehabilitation service, a significant mechanism found to be in operation was the stories that patients told, and the way that these were processed by the health care staff who listened to them. The stories that patients told about themselves, of their experiences of illness and disability, and of their hopes and aspirations were illuminating. In narrating their stories, patients portrayed themselves – implicitly and explicitly – as coping, resourceful, resilient, and creative. The effect that this had on their audience – the health care staff with whom they interact – was to categorize patients in various ways, for example, as 'realistic' or 'unrealistic' or 'in denial'. Listening to these stories, it became apparent that one of the mechanisms at work here was as follows: the way that patients position themselves in the stories that they tell actively contributes to their not getting adequate rehabilitation. In the remainder of this chapter, I will explain what this means. I will start with a discussion of speech act theory to show how stories work, and then go on to apply this to the stories told by two particular patients.

Narrative and story

In explaining how patients as storytellers use a range of devices to achieve particular effects in their listeners, I wish to make clear the distinction between 'narrative' and 'story' (see Paley, this volume), and to be clear that in the context of this analysis, I am referring specifically to stories, with characteristic and identifiable features.

To count as a story, a narrative must meet a number of criteria. First, the causal claims inherent in the narrative must provide an explanation of something. Second, there must be at least one character who is centrally involved in the events described, and this character is confronted with a situation in need of resolution. Third, a link between the central character and the explanation is required, in the sense that the explanation will either account for the character's problem, or show how it is resolved. Finally, the configuration of character, problem, and explanation – in other words, a 'plot' – must be made possible, and will usually be designed to elicit, an emotional reaction from the reader. For example, by portraying the central character in a certain light, the storyteller may arouse the reader's sympathy, disapproval, or admiration. These features meet the criteria set out by Prince (1991: 72), who argues that plot is 'the global dynamic (goal-oriented and forward-moving) organization of narrative constituents which is responsible for the thematic interest ... of a narrative and for its emotional effect'. And it is the organization of narrative constituents responsible for an emotional effect that is essential to the concept of a story, irrespective of whether the story is an account of something that happened, or a work of fiction (for a more in-depth discussion of the relation between 'narrative' and 'story', see Eva and Paley, 2006, and Paley and Eva, 2005).

How stories work: speech act theory

In my analysis of patients' stories, I make use of techniques borrowed from literary criticism to examine the ways in which patients construct narratives in order to create impressions of themselves and others. In doing so, I have assumed that stories are not only accounts of 'how it seems to me' but that they are, much more, accounts of 'how I want it to seem to you'. It is worth noting here that a special case of 'you' is oneself: stories can be as much an exercise in self-persuasion as they are in persuading others.

This idea can be developed by applying speech act theory to stories (Austin, 1975; Bortolussi and Dixon, 2003; Searle, 1979). Austin's central claim is that all modes of speaking and writing are performative. Anything said or written has three dimensions: the locution, the illocution, and the perlocution. The locution is the sense of what is said, the illocution is the act thereby performed, and the perlocution is the effect of the performance. If, for example, I say to somebody, 'You will fall if you're not careful', the 'locution' is what this sentence means. But to utter the sentence is to perform an act: it is to issue a warning. That is the illocutionary force of the sentence; and if, when I give my warning, the other person feels cautious, or worried, or annoyed, that is the perlocution, the *effect* which uttering the sentence has. Take another example: 'I'm sorry I'm late. I stopped to help my neighbour with a flat tyre.' Here the perlocution is to reduce possible irritation at one's tardiness, and this is (arguably) achieved by presenting oneself as a kind, helpful person. The illocution would be to apologize, and offer an excuse. In general terms, other illocutionary acts include naming, praising, questioning, advising, promising, confirming, and of course many more.

To this list we can add narrating and storytelling. Telling a story, whether in spoken or written form, is an illocutionary act, whose perlocutionary force is the emotional cadence (Velleman, 2003) which is in fact produced, and which may well be intended by the storyteller. Stories can, of course, be told purely to entertain; but perlocution is a way of referring to the fact that they are frequently intended to manipulate – not necessarily in a pejorative sense – those who hear them. 'Stories are not innocent', observes Chambers (1984: 7): they have a 'performative function', eliciting audience reaction by means of 'narrative seduction'. One form of narrative analysis, then, is to understand how a story's textual features are processed by the reader in a way that secures this reaction.

How stories work: the need for narrative vigilance

To illustrate the power of stories, I will use – for the sake of brevity and convenience – a very short generic palliative care story written by David Cameron, a doctor who works in rural Southern Africa (Becker, 2005: 52):

> Home-based care? Flies circle like lazy vultures parting the air saturated with the smell of cervical cancer. Too weak to sit up, she reached out and grasped my hand, 33 degrees outside, it felt like 40 under the low tin roof. 'Hospital?' I suggested. 'No, people die there.' Six pairs of weary eyes watch my every move.

This story packs a great deal into its 57 words. To understand how rich the selection of storyworld detail is, we can compare it with an alternative narrative account of the same events:

> On a hot afternoon, I did a home visit to a woman with advanced cancer. I suggested admission to hospital. She declined.

It is obvious that the impact of the story has completely disappeared. The imagery of the original story, unlike the bare narrative of the second version, creates a richly textured world, providing the reader with a strongly sensual awareness of the heat, the smells, the imminence of death. And what of the narrator? What do we make of this doctor's predicament? He is faced with a very sick woman reaching out to him; in the weariness of the woman's family, the rejection of hospital, the inadequacy of home-based care, the evident poverty, there is a sense of exhausted options. We are invited to feel some sympathy for the doctor's burden of responsibility. The first version of the story elicits a response from its audience in a way that the second does not, and that difference is contained in the way that story elements combine to achieve a particular effect.

However brief, then, the story is a powerful one; and that, of course, is the point. Stories, well told and well constructed, trigger an emotional response of some kind, sometimes strong, sometimes subtle. That is why they are told. As a consequence, they can deter analysis, and there is a danger that we will mistake 'emotional closure for intellectual closure' (Velleman, 2003: 20) and fail to acknowledge that a story 'enables its audience to assimilate events, not to familiar patterns of *how things happen,* but rather to familiar patterns of *how things feel*' (Velleman, 2003: 19). This is the seductive quality of stories: they are designed to elicit the perlocutionary effect intended by the author, deter serious analysis, and distract the audience's attention away from the narrative machinery that achieves this very outcome.

Of course, stories *may* be true (or accurately reflect a general truth) as well as emotionally resonant. But, equally, they may not be. It is crucial to distinguish between two different reactions to any story: 'emotionally satisfying' on the one hand, and 'likely to be true' on the other; or, conversely, 'emotionally unsettling', and therefore a 'source of suspicion'. There is a marked tendency for all of us, if we are not careful, to slide from one to the other. Emotionally satisfying (or unsettling) . . . and *therefore* (if only subconsciously) likely to be true (or suspect) (Velleman, 2003). Understanding of how stories 'work' can help us to avoid these slides.

Techniques in literary criticism

I have suggested that narrators deploy a range of narrative devices to achieve – wittingly or unwittingly – a particular effect. I will now describe some of these devices, and go on to show how an analysis of their use in patients' stories can contribute to our understanding of the particular mechanism at work here.

The basic ingredients of stories are well known: they have characters, contexts, plots, beginnings, middles, and ends. Good stories are constructed so that they are coherent. We tend to be more satisfied with stories in which loose ends are tied up, virtue is rewarded, the villains get their come-uppance, and a problem of some kind is resolved. We also like stories which surprise us, which are involving, and those which describe events and circumstances in an immediate, compelling way (Davis, 1987; Hills, 2000). All of these contribute to a story's appeal; by the same token, they invite an emotional engagement with the story, and are, as I have argued, reasons for approaching stories with careful attention.

From the vast range of techniques used in literary criticism I can obviously select only a handful to illustrate their use in practice. I am going to focus on three: plot, characterization, and narrative style in terms of narrator reliability. I am using these as they demonstrate most effectively the interaction between patient-narrator and health-care-professional-listener pertinent to the analysis of the 'little rehabilitation' outcome. However, I am also drawing on aspects such as close reading, comparisons, disjunctions, inconsistencies, and conflict (Abbott, 2002; Manlove, 1989; Miller, 2001; Rimmon-Kenan, 2002).

Plot: the logic of the story

Stories, irrespective of whether they are made up or claim to be about real events, have some kind of plot. In identifying plot in narrative, we are pointing to a kind of unity, the way in which events and characters are linked together into a schematic whole (see Paley, this volume, for a further discussion of plot). We are inclined to connect our thinking about life to a number of masterplots (virtue rewarded, such as this one, or others: a quest, stories of revenge, tales of death and renewal, and so on). As both storytellers and story-hearers, we have a tendency to overlook raw evidence in favour of establishing a satisfactorily coherent plot framework for a story. In effect, plot is a form of generalization; and, in identifying the plot, we assign the narrative to a class of similar stories, with whose contours we are already comfortably familiar.

Characterization

Characters reveal themselves in stories through their actions, their motives, and their thoughts and feelings. Since we can never enter the mind of a character, the best we can do is to infer qualities from clues dispersed throughout the story (Rimmon-Kenan, 2002). A narrator elicits different responses to different characters by the way he or she portrays them, and also invites a response towards himself or herself as narrator.

The way in which the events are narrated, and the way the story is received by the audience, will be shaped by the cultural context in which the story is told, and by the pre-existing preferences of the reader or listener. Individual backgrounds, different experiences, different sets of associations, different fears, different desires can all have an impact on the extent to which we identify with one character or another. Take the example of the story of Cinderella. We are usually invited to identify with the heroine, and to take a dim view of the ugly sisters. But if you grew up as an ungainly, unattractive girl with few friends, and if you had a beautiful little sister who complained incessantly every time anyone asked her to do some modest task around the house, who claimed to be downtrodden and unloved despite the constant attention of a wealthy godmother, and who wound up marrying a prince, then you might see the story in a very different light. The portrayal of character and the perspective from which a story is told interacts with cultural and individual proclivities; and the storyteller, whether consciously or unconsciously, shapes the narrative in such a way as to evoke or trigger these pre-existing preferences and expectations.

Reliable and unreliable narrators

In analysing a story, questions can be asked about the reliability or unreliability of the narrator (Booth, 1961). Where a narrator shares values with the reader (or listener), and appears accurately to observe and record the world, reader rapport and trust is encouraged. However, a narrator who displays a lack of self-awareness, or who appears to have values at odds with the audience, or who recounts events at odds with other evidence, is seen to be unreliable. When hearing or reading stories, the listener or reader will make judgements about the extent to which the narrator can be relied upon for an accurate account, and react accordingly.

Stories told by patients

In the remainder of this chapter, I will contrast the stories told by two patients: Gill and Eddie. For each of their stories, I will show how an analysis of plot, characterization, and narrator reliability gives us a framework for understanding the responses of the rehabilitation staff towards them.

Gill's story

Gill narrated many stories in which she portrayed herself as competent, resilient, capable, and resourceful: how she had prepared for receiving the anticipated news of her initial diagnosis of breast cancer by calling her deputy managers to her hospital bed and giving a thorough handover of work for the coming weeks; her organization of the installation of a custom-built stair lift, where she coordinated the efforts of several health and social services agencies. In the following example, she describes the arrangements she has made for her funeral:

> Everything has been arranged, from a to z. I had the funeral directors around, chose my coffin. I love my husband to death, but I love my mum and dad to death as well. And it did worry me – if get buried here, then it's too far for my mum and dad to come if they're feeling they want to grieve one day, and vice versa, Graham. So I've spoken to both of the vicars who come and visit me, and although I didn't really want to get cremated, I'm going to be cremated, and there are going to be two caskets; one will be buried back home and one will be buried here. I've chosen the hymns, chosen the music I want played – one of the vicars e-mailed me the service with the missing bits I needed to fill in – and it's all done. So if, God forbid, I take a turn for the worse today or tomorrow, the i's are dotted the t's are crossed on the service and what I want.

Let us consider the story being told here. Gill has a problem: her parents' home is several hundred miles away from where Gill lives with her husband, Graham. She loves them all, and knows that they each want a tangible focus for their grief after her death. The basic logic – or plot – is a problem, a dilemma which is solved by a resourceful, problem-solving narrator, hence eliciting the audience's approval. Seeing it against a plot type helps to categorize it, and contributes to shaping – probably quite unconsciously – a response. A puzzle is solved. As a generic plot-type, we could think of Oedipus solving the Sphinx's riddle, or the biblical story of the judgement of Solomon. We are invited to be satisfied at the resolution of a potentially problematic situation, and to be supportive of the action of the central character.

We can see the essential features of this story – those that contribute to an understanding of what this story is about – as Gill's equally strong feelings for husband and parents (she is a loving wife and a loving daughter); the geographical distance between her parents and husband; her preference not to be cremated, but her willingness to set aside her own wishes in order to meet the needs of others (she is both unselfish and practical); her detailed organization of her funeral (she is a planner, resourceful, capable of securing the help of others, like the vicars, when required). All of these elements have to be present for the story to do its work. Through her characterization of herself, we are invited to see her as meticulous, organized, problem-solving, subordinating her wishes to those of her loved ones, and capable of getting help when needed.

Gill portrays herself as a reliable narrator. She tells us that she worried about what she was going to do: this was no whim, no careless spur of the moment fancy. She has considered the matter carefully, decided on a course of action, and made her arrangements.

The health care staff with whom Gill came into contact accepted her account of herself as positive and coping, as these examples show:

> [Occupational therapist] She was remaining incredibly positive considering what was happening to her, the rapid changes and her loss around becoming a paraplegic. We talked about what she was going to be able to manage and what she wasn't going to be able to manage, and my perception was that she was holding it together because that's her personality. She's a professional lady and has always taken a bright outlook on things as far as she can.

> [Social worker] She is a very competent person, and she has overcome a lot of the problems herself, in terms of things like finding somebody to provide the care that she wants. She's very resourceful, she will not sit there feeling sorry for herself. She will sit there working on ways of achieving what she wants.

> [Clinical nurse specialist] Gill's a great initiator. She knows how to take things forward and she's very clear about you don't wait around for people to do stuff for you, you get on and do it yourself.

Gill had a warm relationship with staff. The occupational therapist, for example, had responded quickly and helpfully to her requests for items of equipment – such as the stair lift, and a hoist for the bath – and was very respectful of Gill's wishes and preferences. She describes Gill's discharge home after a stay in the hospice in-patient unit:

> Gill went home adamant that she wanted to be upstairs, which we completely went with because that was her wish. The bath was highly important to her and there was no way of having a bath downstairs, and she felt that was a better option.

I now want to contrast Gill's story with that of Eddie.

Eddie's story

Like Gill, Eddie presented himself as a problem-solver. Here, he is anticipating his discharge home from hospital following radiotherapy treatment:

> Three o'clock in the morning, I'm wide awake and my head's going round just thinking [about home] and what I'm going to do: how I'm going to get the rice pudding from the kitchen to my table. I've got the problem solved. I've got a tea trolley I made. I made a table top for it, we used to play cards on it, and it was just the right size for dinner for two or three. I've also got a six foot long workbench that goes on the top, and that's my workbench for inside with a chair. It's [always had] a dual purpose. Now, the tea trolley, it's got four castors on, [I'll] take back two castors off, build it up, get ordinary piece of wood on the bottom, so that it doesn't slide. I'm sure there's plenty timber down the shed. Make a couple of handles that screw onto the side of the trolley and I can hold on and walk around with the tea trolley. Make it low enough, with the wheels at the front and solid rubber at the back, push, stop, push, stop. Like so. I'm looking forward to going home. It'll be an adventure.

Eddie, too, has a problem: he can't manage to walk with his walking frame and carry things at the same time. He proposes a creative solution: he has a trolley which has already demonstrated its versatility, which he will modify further. Again, a dilemma is solved by a resourceful, problem-solving narrator; however, the plot of Eddie's story is not so much one of careful planning, wisdom, and pragmatism (as Gill's was), but more of adventurous good fortune. This becomes even more evident if we set Eddie's tea-trolley story against a story he told about his life experiences:

> I had a happy childhood. We just ran wild. I used to go and see the blacksmith and watch him pump his bellows when I was seven. I learned more in that fitting shop there, when I did get a job at the factory at fourteen I knew more than the other young starters. As much as I could have done, so I did really well. Fortunately – everything is just fortunately – I meet a good gang of kids, they didn't go drink, they were really good lads. The chaps at work, I was always put in to work with the best ones, I don't know why, but everything seemed to work out right for me. A friend knew someone in the merchant navy, helped me get a job there. I've been to practically every country in the world. The blokes on there were really good fellows, took care of me.

Eddie characterized himself as adventurous, lucky, resourceful, popular, a survivor, someone who is capable of solving his own problems. In both his childhood and adult life, he has had opportunities and good luck. Things had worked out well for him in the past, and we are invited to believe, along with him, that they will continue to do so in the future.

The response elicited

There are some interesting differences both in content and consequences between Eddie's and Gill's stories. Whereas Gill's characterization of herself reassures staff – here is someone who will sensibly manage her affairs – Eddie's does not. The stories that Eddie tells cause alarm. In Gill's account, we can see careful planning, wisdom and pragmatism, but in Eddie's we have something more akin to adventurous good fortune. Gill is seen as a reliable narrator; Eddie is not. His stories blur the boundary between past triumphs and his present situation. For example, it had been some years since he rode a bicycle; however, his use of the present tense in beginning and ending this story serves to frame an event which occurred 60 years previously into his current perspective:

> And I ride a bike, don't I? Another chap and I had a tandem between us. And we used to do about 140 to 150 miles on a Sunday. We came down from Northumberland once, we were invited down to London for a holiday. We set off about quarter past four on the Saturday and we got there about quarter past five on the Sunday afternoon. One day. Overnight. Didn't sleep. No, just straight through the night. I've been keeping fit all my life.

Similarly, with his plans to adapt his tea-trolley, Eddie draws on past skills and capacities to make future plans, appearing to avoid the recognition of any change in his abilities. One can compare Eddie's luck and good fortune: 'fortunately, everything is just fortunately . . .' and 'I don't know why, but everything seemed to work out right for me', with Gill's much more grounded account: 'everything has been arranged, from a to z', 'the i's are dotted the t's are crossed'. Unlike Eddie, Gill is not leaving matters to chance; her arrangements have been made. Gill's altruism (her concern for her family) resonates with values of the palliative care health professionals; Eddie's buccaneering spirit, conflicting as it does with his audience's concerns for safety, creates anxiety.

In consequence, the responses of the health care professionals are very different in Eddie's case. The occupational therapist notes a change in Eddie's outlook over time, perceiving him to become less and less willing to compromise:

> [When I first met him] he was relatively realistic, saying that he didn't think that he would cope at home as he was. I agreed that he needed to be independent with his transfers and mobility before he could go home. But he didn't really improve with radiotherapy and he was getting more and more frustrated, maybe he felt like we were handling him with kid gloves a little bit, saying you know you're not ready to go home. The more conversations I had with him, the less he seemed to understand what we were getting at and that he wouldn't be able to go back to how he was originally. Eventually we said you've got options: either go home as you are but agree not to undertake any kitchen activities, or if you want to maintain your independence then we need to maybe make adaptations to the kitchen. He was saying that he just needed a rail on the work surface, things that we thought maybe weren't so appropriate because work surfaces aren't really supposed to be used for such weight bearing activities.

The more that staff reject Eddie's notions of himself as resourceful and capable, the more entrenched he becomes in his position. Eddie's determination to hold onto his sense of himself as capable and independent causes the occupational therapist to oppose him even more firmly, not recognizing that her contradiction of his perception of himself contributes to his dismissal of her help. Her response to his ongoing efforts to persuade her of his competence is to oppose him even more firmly:

> We had to be quite assertive with him to make him understand where we were coming from and why we were saying what we were saying. [. . .] I think he sees himself as a very able man and very independent and really wanted to maintain that throughout which was difficult really for us then, because we were trying – in a way we were taking away his independence by recommending care to go home with, saying that he would get home sooner if he would accept those sort of things.

The occupational therapist's concern about Eddie's account of himself can be contrasted with the staff's response to Gill. Gill's characterization of herself is not questioned: 'she *is* a very competent person', 'she *is* very resourceful', 'she *is* a great initiator', whereas Eddie is not seen to be reliable: 'he *sees himself as* a very able man'. Gill's wish to remain upstairs in her home was supported – 'she went home adamant that she wanted to be upstairs, which we completely went with because that was her wish' – but Eddie's ideas are rejected: 'he was saying that he just needed a rail on the work surface, things that we thought maybe weren't so appropriate'.

Eddie received a great deal of attention from the rehabilitation staff and from social services in planning his discharge, and welcomed none of it. He grudgingly accepted what staff said he had to have in order to be allowed home, and refused all community rehabilitation follow-up offered:

> [Occupational therapist] I asked him whether he wanted me to make a referral to the [community services] for ongoing rehab at home because I knew independence was really important to him. He declined a referral which was a bit of a shame really but he said that he'd had enough people going in. I tried to explain that it wasn't a matter of them visiting him it was a matter of carrying on the work that we were doing in hospital at home. [. . .] I was really surprised actually, I really thought, he'd be very keen on that.

Eddie struggled at home for two weeks before being re-admitted through the accident and emergency department to a general medical ward, where he died a few weeks later.

We can see here the way in which the increasing tension between Eddie's view of himself as competent, and the occupational therapist's sense of him as anything but, contributed significantly to Eddie receiving very little rehabilitation. Returning to Gill's situation, we have a different dynamic, but essentially the same outcome in terms of the provision of rehabilitation. Like Eddie, Gill received very little meaningful help with managing disability. Gill, as we have seen, was well organized, adept at eliciting help from numerous individuals and agencies, communicating to staff the message: 'I'll be fine.' In the event, however, she found herself struggling. Here, for example, is her account of the first time she went out of her home in a wheelchair:

> The first time I used it, it was the wrong move really, because we went to [the supermarket] and it was busy, and there I was down in this wheelchair and all of these people, I just felt all these people coming towards me. And it was like – oh, I had no control. It was terrifying, absolutely terrifying and I just wanted to get out.

In Eddie's case, the staff's rejection of his account of himself as competent led to him refusing rehabilitation; in Gill's case, their acceptance of her as capable and resourceful meant that interventions beyond the basic provision of equipment were not offered. The installation of a stair lift and the provision of a wheelchair became ends in themselves, with no further exploration of what they could be instrumental in helping her to achieve.

Conclusion

In this chapter, I have suggested that the way in which health care staff 'process' patients' narratives leads them to make various assumptions, which in turn lead to various decisions. This 'processing' is based on the cues which the narrative itself provides, and it is a key mechanism, in this case, in the inadequate provision of rehabilitation for patients with metastatic spinal cord compression. A careful examination of these cues – the range of narrative features and devices that stories employ – can provide an understanding of the causal link between story and response. If we can trace how the features of a story – such as plot, characterization, and narration – encourage the 'audience' to 'read' it in a particular way, we can understand why the audience then reacts as it does.

A remarkably similar feature of the patients' narratives in this study of a rehabilitation service, was their portrayal of themselves as resourceful, resilient, problem-solving, organized, able to cope with situations that might have defeated others: 'Yes, there are problems,' they would say in effect, 'but I've got them all worked out.' This way of presenting themselves had one of two consequences, depending in part on whether their audience (the staff with whom they came into contact) judged them to be reliable or unreliable narrators. Where patients managed to convey the impression of themselves as trustworthy, their message of 'I'm a capable person,' gained the response of, 'That's fine then, you don't need our help,' and rehabilitation beyond the provision of aids and equipment was not forthcoming. However, where the 'I'm coping,' message was doubted, interventions to ensure physical safety were insisted upon. Usually these met with outright resistance from patients who, after all, believed that they had things under control, and could not see the need for the fuss, bother and intrusion.

In telling stories, patients exploit linguistic, psychological, and cultural resources to generate a particular emotional reaction. There is a link between how a story is structured and our emotional response to it. Equally, there is a range of ways in which we can be invited to identify with, or distance ourselves from, one or more of the characters. The overall effect, then, is to produce a pattern which ties the narrated events together, and which at the same time connects them to a corresponding pattern of emotion.

The patients' portrayal of themselves as resourceful and resilient makes a crucial difference, either because they appear not to need rehabilitation (so are not offered any), or because they do not see themselves as needing it (so reject it when it is offered). There is a deep irony in this, because while hope, optimism, and an ability to view the future positively are desirable in achieving a good quality of life, it turns out to be the patients' demonstration of these very qualities that leads to rehabilitation not being provided.

An awareness of this dynamic, and a willingness not to take stories at face value could contribute to health care staff's ability to recognize that they need to respect and support patients' presentation of self as resourceful, while at the same time finding more oblique ways of 'nudging' patients towards behaviours that would enable a level of participation in daily life which would safeguard psychological and physical well-being.

References

Abbott, H. P. (2002) *The Cambridge Introduction to Narrative*. Cambridge University Press, Cambridge.

Austin, J. L. (1975) *How to Do Things with Words* (2nd edn). Harvard University Press, Cambridge.

Barnard, D., Towers, A. M., Boston, P., and Lambrinidou, Y. (2000) *Crossing Over: Narratives of Palliative Care*. Oxford University Press, Oxford.

Becker, R. (2005) Short stories (editorial). *International Journal of Palliative Nursing*, **11**, 52.

Booth, W. C. (1961) *The Rhetoric of Fiction*. University of Chicago Press, Chicago.

Bortolussi, M., and Dixon, P. (2003) *Psychonarratology: Foundations for the Empirical Study of Literary Response*. Cambridge University Press, Cambridge.

Catz, A., Goldin, D., Fishel, B., Ronen, J., Bluvshtein, V., and Gelernter, I. (2004) Recovery of neurologic function following nontraumatic spinal cord lesions in Israel. *Spine*, **29**(20), 2278–82.

Chambers, R. (1984) *Story and Situation: Narrative Seduction and the Power of Fiction.* Manchester University Press, Manchester.

Cowap, J., Hardy, J. R., and A'Hern, R. (2000) Outcome of malignant spinal cord compression at a cancer centre: implications for palliative care services. *Journal of Pain and Symptom Management*, **19**(4), 257–64.

Davis, L. J. (1987) *Resisting Novels: Ideology and Fiction*. Methuen, London.

Devery, K. (2006) The framework for evidence in palliative care: narrative-based evidence. *Palliative Medicine*, **20**(1), 5.

Elster, J. (1989) *Nuts and Bolts for the Social Sciences*. Cambridge University Press, Cambridge.

Eriks, I, E., Angenot, E. L. D., and Lankhorst, G. J. (2004) Epidural metastatic spinal cord compression: functional outcome and survival after inpatient rehabilitation. *Spinal Cord*, **42**, 235–39.

Eva, G. (2006) *Spinal Cord Compression Secondary to Cancer: Disability and Rehabilitation*. Sir Michael Sobell House, Oxford.

Eva, G. (2007) Spinal Cord Compression Secondary to Cancer: Disability and Rehabilitation. Unpublished PhD Thesis. University of Stirling.

Eva, G. and Paley, J. (2006) Stories in palliative care. *Progress in Palliative Care*, **14**(4), 155–64.

Frank, A. W. (2000) Illness and autobiographical work: dialogue as narrative destabiliza-tion. *Qualitative Sociology*, **23**(1), 135–56.

Greenhalgh, T. and Hurwitz, B. (1998) *Narrative Based Medicine: Dialogue and Discourse in Clinical Practice*. BMJ Books, London.

Guo, Y., Young, B., Palmer, J. L., Mun, Y., and Bruera, E. (2003) Prognostic factors for sur-vival in metastatic spinal cord compression. A retrospective study in a rehabilitation setting. *American Journal of Physical Medicine and Rehabilitation*, **82**(9), 665–68.

Hills, R. (2000) *Writing in General and the Short Story in Particular*. Boston: Mariner Books.

Hurwitz, B., Greenhalgh, T., and Skultans, V. (2002) *Narrative Research in Health and Illness*. BMJ Books, London.

Kirshblum, S., O'Dell, M. W., Ho, C., and Barr, K. (2001) Rehabilitation of persons with central nervous system tumours. *Cancer*, **92**(4 Suppl), 1029–38.

Maddocks, I. (2003) Clinical exegesis and narrative medicine. *Progress in Palliative Care*, **11**(1), 1–2.

Manlove, C. (1989) *Critical Thinking. A Guide to Interpreting Literary Texts*. Macmillan, Basingstoke.

McKinley, W. O., Seel, R. T., and Hardman, J. T. (1999) Nontraumatic spinal cord injury: incidence, epidemiology and functional outcome. *Archives of Physical Medicine and Rehabilitation*, **80**, 619–23.

Miller, L. (2001) *Mastering Practical Criticism*. Palgrave, Basingstoke.

Paley, J., and Eva, G. (2005) Narrative vigilance: the analysis of stories in health care. *Nursing Philosophy*, **6**(2), 83–97.

Pawson, R., and Tilley, N. (1997) *Realistic Evaluation*. Sage, London.

Prince, G. (1991) *Dictionary of Narratology*. Scolar Press, Aldershot.

Quill, T. E. (1996) *A Midwife Through the Dying Process: Stories of Healing and Hard Choices at the End of Life*. Johns Hopkins University Press, Baltimore.

Rimmon-Kenan, S. (2002) *Narrative Fiction* (2nd edn). Routledge, London.

Searle, J. (1979) *Expression and Meaning: Studies in the Theory of Speech Acts*. Cambridge University Press, Cambridge.

Tang, V., Harvey, D., Park Dorsay, J., Jiang, S., and Rathbone, M. P. (2007) Prognostic indicators in metastatic spinal cord compression: using functional independence measure and Tokuhashi scale to optimize rehabilitation planning. *Spinal Cord,* **45**(10), 671–77.

Velleman, J. D. (2003) Narrative explanation. *Philosophical Review,* **112**, 1–25.

Chapter 7

Narrative and storytelling in palliative care education and training

Karen Forbes

This chapter explores how narrative and storytelling are being used in education and training, and how these approaches have, or could be, used in teaching and learning in palliative care. I will draw on examples from my own teaching. As a doctor these examples will be related to teaching medical students and doctors. However, the chapter will also engage with education and training for other health care professionals, particularly nurses.

Histories and the novice practitioner

Health care is a storied world. During our first consultation we ask the patient to tell us their story. Students are trained to take a 'history', a process of inter-rogating, reducing and refining a patient's story into a structure which has undoubted utility in suggesting a disease or diagnosis, but which may strip away, or at least afford less importance to the person's lived experience of that diagnosis or disease. Students are trained to see the patient's disease through a particular lens, but in doing so may miss the stories which tell of the illness, characterized as the sick person's experience (Kleinman, 1988). The current 'turn to narrative' urges us to broaden or even turn away from the positivist stance we have been trained into, so that we might learn 'how to encompass in our minds the complexity of some lived moments in life' (Coles, 1989: 128). Coles, a physician, argues 'you don't do that with theories. You don't do that with a system of ideas. You do it with a story' (Coles, 1989: 128). Narrative, it is argued, 'provides meaning, context and perspective for the patient's predica-ment'. It 'offers a possibility of developing an understanding [of the illness experience] that cannot be arrived at by any other means' (Greenhalgh and Hurwitz 1999: 325).

While learning to take a 'history' may be reductive, this approach may be necessary because of the sheer volume of knowledge and skills that have to be acquired by the novice practitioner. To walk onto a ward as a junior medical student, for example, is to enter an established organization as a stranger, not knowing the rules and fearful of breaking them. To approach a patient who is ill, perhaps afraid, and 'take a (medical) history' can be overwhelming. Instead, students are asked to 'go and talk to a patient'. This helps them get over their initial hesitation about approaching people by asking them to do something they can do, which is 'just' talk to them. These students come away with rich, multilayered stories about the person's disease, certainly, but also about their lives and families, and often their hopes and fears. They learn that they can talk to patients, and often gain new perspectives about people from different generations, cultures and classes from their own. Two or three years later this same student will be proficient in taking a 'polished' medical history, stripped of 'extraneous' detail. However, while a focused medical history can be criticized as not being 'holistic', it fulfils a number of functions: first, the student learns to recognize the patterns of symptoms which come together in particular illnesses; secondly it helps the student to organize what can be a jumble of information into a manageable form, to identify priorities and therefore direct best patient care; and thirdly, it can enable a swift and accurate diagnosis, which can be a matter of life and death.

The structured, somewhat bare narrative that is a health care history may omit the detail that makes the patient recounting that history an individual, and can therefore be criticized as distancing students or qualified practitioners from those they interact with. While this criticism might be justified at times, established advanced practitioners should remember how overwhelming coming into contact with illness, suffering, dying and death on a daily basis is for the novice practitioner, and recognize that some distancing is necessary for that novice to endure, learn and grow within such an environment. However, Kleinman suggests that this 'bare' history:

> encourage[s physicians] to believe that *disease* is more important than *illness*, that all they need is knowledge about biology, not knowledge about the psychosocial and cultural aspects of illness. . . . The gauntlet of residency training may even dehumanize the practitioner, and certainly does not contribute to the training of physicians committed to psychosocially sensitive care.
>
> (Kleinman, 1988: 255–6)

Inui and Frankel suggest that this tendency to see the patient with *disease* rather than the person suffering *illness*, and the maintenance of distance between the patient and the professional might be because patients are strangers to us:

> The people with whom we interact daily are often strangers, very different from ourselves. They are sick, we are healthy. They are weak, and we are strong. They act in unaccountable ways and are desperate, afraid, or sometimes abusive. They are old

when we are young and young when we are old. They speak different languages, recognize other gods, and see the world working in ways peculiar to us.

(Inui and Frankel, 2006: 415)

Inui and Frankel argue that we need approaches – humanistic medicine, patient-centred medicine, relationship centred medicine – 'founded on understanding what it takes to respond constructively and whole-heartedly to strangers, both to patients and to [the stranger within] our innermost selves' (p. 416).

To take a history is thus to funnel our enquiry towards an important end; however, in order to engage with the complexity of Coles' (1989) 'lived moments' in the strangers we encounter, we need to avoid discarding those narratives and stories that appear superfluous to our diagnostic goal; rather, to see them as complementary, enriching and necessary to achieving best patient care. In the following section I will outline some of the ways that narrative and storytelling are being used in education and training to achieve this end.

Narrative medicine and narrative competence

The origins and definition of narrative medicine and narrative techniques used to support clinical practice are discussed in Chapter 2. Many medical authors have argued that the lost tradition of narrative should be revived in the teaching and practice of medicine so that doctors can better relate to and understand the patient's perspective and story (Elwyn and Gwyn, 1999; Greenhalgh, 1999; Greenhalgh and Hurwitz, 1999; Launer, 1999).

Charon, a strong promoter of narrative medicine, advocates the development of 'narrative competence' in medicine (Chapter 2 provides a further elaboration of narrative competence), and suggests that this can be achieved through writing and the study of literature (Charon, 2000a). She argues that the study of literature can 'help doctors understand what happens in patients' lives . . . increase doctors' and medical students' narrative competence . . . develop skills in accurately interpreting the texts of medicine [and] help doctors to develop the capacity for self-knowledge and reflection' (Charon, 2000b: 285). For Charon, literary competence teaches and mirrors narrative competence in medicine, so the student or doctor can pay attention to the form, plot, and chronology of the story offered and learn to listen both to what is said and not said. The reader (or listener) learns to tolerate uncertainty and ambiguity and becomes curious about what is happening in the story and their own reactions to it. Literary competence 'calls for the exercise of skill in observation and interpretation, develops clinical imagination, and, especially through writing, preserves fluency in ordinary language and promotes clarity of observation, expression, and self-knowledge' (Hunter et al. 1995: 787). The difference between a story listened to by a narratively competent practitioner and a medical 'history' lies in an openness to listen to the person's 'whole' story, without prematurely honing in on diagnostic clues, risking cutting out the patient's experience.

Charon's students keep 'parallel charts' on their patients during their internal medicine attachments. While they record the patients' clinical findings, observations and results of investigations in the conventional chart or patient's notes, they record their communication with the patient and family, and their feelings and reflections about being involved in the patient's care in their parallel chart. Once a week they bring and read out something from their parallel chart to a small group meeting. Charon uses the skills of literary criticism to observe and interrogate the structure of the piece presented. She has gained funding to examine the effects of such writing and reading on the way that doctors learn and subsequently practise. Preliminary results indicate that students allocated randomly to keep parallel charts are more able to interact with patients and their families and both their clinical and communication skills are rated more highly by their tutors than those students completing a 'standard' medical clerkship (Charon, 2004). Using a similar writing and reading approach within a 'Healing Narratives' course, Sierpina and colleagues advocate 'making' rather than 'taking' a history, so that, through 'coconstruct[ing] with the patient the reality of the medical encounter and the tone and timbre of the healing relationship' students can learn a 'new kind of relationship-centred, patient-centred care model' (Sierpina et al. 2007: 626).

Narrative and storytelling in reflective practice

While Charon and Sierpina argue for narrative competence as a way of teaching holistic history 'making', many authors argue that the role of narrative and storytelling in health care education is to facilitate reflective practice. Evidence-based practice and reflective practice are often presented as diametrically opposed approaches, in my view unfairly. The proponents of evidence-based medicine always advocated careful clinical judgement as to whether the available evidence was applicable to the particular patient:

> Knowing the tools of evidence-based practice is necessary but not sufficient for delivering the highest quality patient care. In addition to clinical expertise, the clinician requires compassion, sensitive listening skills, and broad perspectives from the humanities and social sciences. These attributes allow understanding of patients' illnesses in the context of their experience, personalities and cultures.
>
> (Guyatt et al. 2000: 1293)

It is argued that these attributes can be gained through reflection, 'the process of internally examining and exploring issues of concern, triggered by experience, which creates and clarifies meaning in terms of self, and which results in a changed conceptual perspective' (Boyd and Fales, 1983: 100).

Schön argues that reflecting during (reflection-in-action) and after (reflection-on-action) 'situations of practice [which are] not problems to be solved but problematic situations characterized by uncertainty, disorder and indeterminacy' allows us to respond to these 'messy, confusing problems [which] defy technical solution' (Schön, 1983: 3). It is held that storytelling as an aid to reflection can increase understanding and appreciation of the patient's lived experience, enhance self-esteem, encourage critical thinking and increase knowledge and communication skills, cultural and ethical sensitivity and role-model hope and strength (Davidhizar and Lonser, 2003).

Storytelling can also foster listening (to the whole story and not just its parts), partnership (encouraging collaboration between the professional and the patient), reciprocity (when stories are shared both learning and teaching occurs, increasing mutual respect), and solidarity (a joining together through exchange of ideas and beliefs). It is argued these aims can be met through many forms of storytelling, including case studies, journals, stories from practice, life reviews and reminiscence (Schwartz and Abbott, 2007).

While the learning facilitated by reflection is often memorable and important, the process of telling stories can make the narrator vulnerable, and hence providing a safe, confidential space in which stories can be shared is critical. If this 'safe space' can be created, however, sharing narratives can enable students and practitioners genuinely to learn from their reflections (Levett-Jones, 2007).

There are many instances of storytelling as an aid to reflection, particularly in the nursing literature, and only a few examples can be presented here. Hunter and Hunter (2006) invited students to present stories about midwifery practice during a weekly midwifery course. Stories allowed students to recognize that they were experiencing similar achievements and frustrations to others. They valued being 'able to process a clinical situation with group feedback and support, which, in turn, provided personal growth and further self-reflection' (Hunter and Hunter, 2006: 275). Students gained cognitive learning, emotional clarification about clinical practice and assistance in role transition.

DasGupta (2003) describes facilitating humanities seminars for medical students called 'Reading the Body, Writing the Body: Women's Illness Narratives' to investigate gender. Students studied literature by women about women and critiqued women's illness narratives, as well as writing, reflecting upon and refining their own. DasGupta concludes that medical students may be 'coerced by the medical establishment to abandon the needs of their bodies in favour of their minds. But it is a mere punctuation – a comma, a breath, a course, a reading, a paragraph written – that separates them from their very real and varied bodies'. This 'physician disembodiment' should be addressed by 'writing, speaking, teaching and discussing . . . the lesson learned in patient narratives [to] make it our own' (DasGupta, 2003: 251). This article is recommended as a resource because the structure of the six-week course, the writing assignments and the rich and varied reading suggested are included in the appendix. Other authors have used storytelling to encourage students to assess cultural needs (Evans and Severtsen, 2001) and to explore 'uncertain, impossible, ambiguous [clinical] situations' (Belling, 2006: 13).

Narrative in professional development

The approaches and courses described above are all for early-career practitioners. Narrative and story can also be used for professional development in established practitioners. Bolton (1999) describes reflective writing groups in postgraduate medical and nursing education in the United Kingdom, some run as part of postgraduate degree courses. Participants write for a short period of time, without planning, on a subject chosen at the meeting. They have time to reflect upon their own writing and whether to share it; the group then discusses portions of this writing and the issues raised. These groups are not therapeutic, although personal issues may be explored. Bolton argues that writing allows participants to reflect, review, and consider when to share, so that 'the writer can afford to say more to the silent page', thus writing 'has a far deeper reflective and educative function' (Bolton, 1999: 244). Participants suggest that such writing groups have enabled them to reach greater depths of professional and personal understanding and have also decreased professional isolation.

Action research

Action research is a 'participatory, democratic process concerned with developing practical knowing. . . . It brings together action and reflection, theory and practice, in participation with others, in the pursuit of practical solutions to issues of pressing concern to people . . . and their communities' (Reason and Bradbury, 2001: 1). There are various methods of action research; they all involve a participatory, cyclical process of action, data gathering, reflection and further action to facilitate change (Fig. 7.1). Fundamental to action research is the generation of new knowledge.

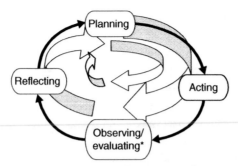

Fig. 7.1 The action research spiral. Adapted with permission of University of Southampton.
* The place of narrative and storytelling in gathering data
Source: Adapted from www.rdsu.soton.ac.uk/documents/Action_research_newsletter.doc

Action research is primarily a research process, however teaching and learning are central to its process and some authors assert that the spirit of collaboration and inquiry applies 'equally well to the classroom' (Schneider and Caswell, 2003: 4).

Appreciative inquiry

While most action research methods are based on problem-solving, appreciative inquiry is influenced by Gergen's (1999) work on social constructionism and the use of language to foster appreciation and understanding. It sees the identification of problems as inherently negative, focusing instead on what is positive about a person or team's practice, circumstances or organization. Storytelling and narrative are central to the initial 'discovery' phase of the four-phase approach; discovery, dream, design, destiny. Appreciative interviews are used to 'discover' stories about the best of *what is* within the organization by focusing participants (storytellers) on a situation when they were functioning at their very best. These stories are used to encourage people, individually and collectively, to 'dream' *what might be*. The 'design' phase challenges participants to determine *what should be*, and to decide upon the organization's 'destiny'; *what will be*. Stories, past, present, and future, and the learning acquired through telling and hearing them, are central to the method.

While appreciative inquiry originated in organizational development (Cooperrider, 1990), it has since been used in a variety of educational and health care settings. Carter (2006) describes how appreciative inquiry has been used in studies about discharge planning for older people, midwives' views of practice in midwifery, and her own work on services for children with complex needs. In an article entitled 'Kicking Eeyore into touch' she advocates appreciative inquiry as one way to encourage nurses to 'celebrate what they do well and embrace and engage with the energy and creativity that underpins strong, resourceful, innovative and expert practice' to 'encourage us to "think solutions"' (Carter, 2007: 181).

In an effort to 'co-create high quality modern patient-centred healthcare' Wright and colleagues describe an appreciative inquiry project on a UK national paediatric liver ward (Wright and Barker, 2005). They wished to 'find out what works, and infuse more of it into the organization's performances'. During the 'discovery' phase of the project, participants were asked for stories about when a patient, parent or family received health care at its best or when they made the difference to what happened in a situation. The authors comment on the 'rich and defining' quality of the stories gathered; of supporting patients and families at times of distress, and of 'making other professionals act to prevent a disaster'. Absence due to sickness was high on the unit, and fell during the project. Two years later many recalled the interviews affecting them profoundly and significantly, usually positively. The authors conclude that these conversations allowed the creation of new, shared possibilities, and encouraged managers to be part of the modernization process, so that all parts of the organization learned and developed.

Narrative and storytelling in developing professionalism

We tell stories to explain our lives, and these stories come together or 'accrue' until 'the accruals eventually create something variously called a "culture" or a "history" or, more loosely, a "tradition"' (Bruner, 1991: 18). Narrative and stories defining such cultures, often as part of action research projects, have been influential in the 'professionalisation, defined as the achievement of autonomous practice and the possession of a discrete body of knowledge', of various roles, notably teaching and nursing (Hart, 1996: 459). 'Professionalising' action research has three components: education (through reflective practice); delineation of problems; and strategies for improvement and involvement. Hart argues that Schön's reflection-in-action produces narrative accounts of a body of professional knowledge that are relevant to nursing practice and foster professional development and social transformation.

In the 'established' profession of medicine, there is much debate about the teaching of medical professionalism, because of a widespread feeling that commitment to professional values is being lost (Inui, 2003). Coulehan (2007) suggests substituting narrative-based professionalism for rule-based professionalism, where the former refers 'to that tradition that values, beliefs and community are essential to medical professionalism . . . For medical professionalism to mould the behaviour of physicians in training, it must be formulated as a meta-narrative – a summation of, and reflection upon, many thousands of actual physicians' stories from different times and cultures' (p. 106). He argues for role modelling through the study of literature written by and about doctors, but also for those portrayed through other media, such as film.

Narrative and storytelling in palliative care education in the literature

Examples of narrative and storytelling in education and training in palliative and end-of-life care are not widespread in the literature. Most use storytelling as a teaching and learning tool, to facilitate reflective practice, or within action research projects.

During the evolution of a graduate course on end-of-life care the premise of the interdisciplinary faculty planning the course was that 'dying . . . is not only a biologic[al] and narrative experience but also a social and cultural process (Myers Schim and Raspa, 2007: 202). They therefore used a narrative and cultural focus to design a course around 15 'story domains', such as physical stories, spiritual stories, ethical/moral stories, and the like. As the course developed each story domain became less discipline specific and more likely to be led by an interdisciplinary team, or by presenters outside their traditional areas. Patients, their carers and families were also involved as teachers. The course is now listed in five university departments as diverse as nursing and anthropology, illustrating its place in encouraging collaboration in professional education.

In an action research project in Australia, experienced palliative care nurses recounted practice stories demonstrating the role of nurse idealism in patient care. While idealism was felt to encourage palliative care nurses to strive for the best for patients, they acknowledged that it could lead them to wish to 'fix everything'. Sharing and reflecting upon stories allowed nurses to improve their practice by acknowledging realistic goals rather than idealistic wishes for perfectionism (Taylor et al. 2002).

In an exemplar of an action research project Hockley and Froggatt (2006) describe how the narratives gained through focus groups, interviews, and collaborative learning groups enabled staff in two nursing homes to explore and develop palliative care knowledge, including adapting and implementing the Liverpool Care Pathway for the Dying (Ellershaw and Wilkinson, 2003) in one of the homes. The article documenting the process is meticulous in explaining the theory behind the study, the collaboration between researchers and staff, the ethical, power and confidentiality issues raised through this collaboration and the importance of reflection and reflexivity throughout.

The authors observe that 'being eclectic and drawing on the different approaches of action research . . . requires considerable knowledge and experience of action research' (p. 836). This can make the practicalities of how reflection can change practice through action research difficult to grasp; the article goes a long way to bridging that 'theory-practice gap'.

In Bolton's work with reflective writing groups death was both a common theme and a 'problem':

> Death is always associated with guilt, grief, pain, fear, anger, disbelief, denial, hopelessness, and only occasionally acceptance. The practitioner's own mortality, and often that of their loved ones, always stares them in the face, as does their (generally unwarranted and irrational) sense of guilt.
>
> (Bolton, 1999: 244)

Discussing death through sharing stories allowed practitioners to compare similar experiences and to reflect upon how patients, families and carers, professional and non-professional, might have felt, the ethical issues raised and what they might have done differently. Bolton suggests that 'we are our stories; writing and rewriting them keeps us alert, alive and flexible. Writing and sharing stories . . . keeps us questioning: medical practice, our patients, ourselves' (Bolton, 1999: 245).

Narrative and storytelling in teaching

I believe our responsibility as teachers of palliative care is to help students understand why palliative care principles matter and how they can use them to improve their care of all patients. I use stories within my teaching to make evidence come alive and to demonstrate its relevance to real people in real situations. Stories can break up didactic teaching, provide a change of focus, demonstrate the application of principles, bridge the theory–practice gap, but also demonstrate the compassion and humanity of patients and professionals. Not even experienced clinicians get things right all of the time and stories can help to counter the predominance of the 'death as failure' narrative (see also DasGupta, Irvine and Spiegel, this volume).

I have used reflective writing in tutorial groups with undergraduate and Masters students. I ask students to write about a memorable patient or 'a patient I have seen this week'. Not all students engage with the task; undoubt-edly some are not ready to make themselves potentially vulnerable. However, my experience echoes that of Charon when she reports:

> students write astonishing prose about anger, sadness, mourning, helplessness, and guilt as well as about victory and accomplishment. When they read to one another,

in small groups, what they have written, they realize they are not isolated in their profound reactions to patient care but that they can talk with their colleagues and their teacher about their reactions to caring for sick patients.

(Charon, 2000b: 289)

In my experience both undergraduate and postgraduate students are surprised by their own writing, about what they and others see within it, and can gain valuable insights into their own and others' responses to caring for sick and dying people.

I also use narrative in a lecture theatre setting within a symposium called 'Dealing with Death'. This is the story of that teaching:

I am standing at the front of a poorly lit, tiered lecture theatre. There are 150 fifth-year medical students stretching away from me. My heart is thumping. I am teaching with Nigel, a consultant in accident and emergency medicine. We begin.

Karen: 'We are going to talk to you as our colleagues, having talked to the parents of a 23 year old student who has died. I am a consultant in Palliative Medicine. I have known Jenny for six months. She had an osteosarcoma diagnosed a year ago, when she was 22. About six weeks ago her chemotherapy was stopped because of disease progression. She was increasingly weak and frail over the last two weeks and had to come into hospital because of breathlessness. When her chemotherapy was stopped I talked to Jenny, her boyfriend and her family with one of our specialist nurses about how ill she was. They all understood she was dying, and she had made preparations for her death, including making plans for her funeral. Jenny deteriorated and died quite quickly. Her family had been called in, but they didn't get to the hospital in time, so I had to tell them she had died. I knew they had been prepared for her death, but I wasn't sure how they would react.

Nigel: 'I am a consultant in Accident and Emergency Medicine. Harry was brought in to A&E after a cycling accident. He was 23. We had been trying to resuscitate him for 40 minutes. The attempt was unsuccessful. My link nurse told me the parents and his brother were in the relatives' room and they had no idea what was going on. I walked towards the door. I had ten yards of preparation time.

We continue, alternating back and forth, giving the next bit of each story, demonstrating, we hope, that the underlying principles of looking after patients and breaking the news of a patient's death are the same, despite the very different care settings. As we begin, we are standing about six metres apart. As we swap from one speaker to another we move gradually so we are standing next to each other as we finish.

This teaching is delivered to fifth-year medical students. We do not introduce the session, we simply begin. Each time one of us falters, each time the room is completely silent, each time I look up briefly and scan faces, each time I see tears. Twice someone has retreated from the room, sobbing. We timetable the afternoon so that I move straight into the next section and Nigel is available to go out after anyone who has left. They have always come back into the lecture theatre, with support from their friends and Nigel.

This is a difficult afternoon. We talk about diagnosing death, death certification, organ transplantation; the end of the timetable reads 'A star, and a postscript'. The star is a man who tells his story of years on dialysis, of looking at his hands the morning after his first renal transplant and realizing they were pink, not yellow; of his transplant failing some years and two children later and having to go back on dialysis, of receiving a second kidney from his wife. I tell the students David will never claim travel expenses for coming to talk to us. He says it is his way of saying thank you. He is warm and candid and funny and very much alive. He is the star.

And the postscript? The postscript goes thus:

> Before we finish I want to give you the Government Health Warning. Standard teaching would be that we should have warned you this afternoon might be distressing and invited you to leave if you wished. We didn't do that. We know that many of you will be dealing with bereavement or someone close to you who is ill. We know we have distressed some of you and for that we apologize. But . . . you are going to be doctors. You are going to look after very sick people; some of them will die. We are sincerely sorry if we have distressed you, but I would rather you were distressed now, amongst your friends and peers, than confronting these issues for the first time with a dying patient in front of you. Please think about how you deal with these issues, and know where your support comes from. Please contact us if you wish to talk about this . . . you know where we are.

This teaching is risky. I know it should be delivered in small groups, but there is no possible time in the curriculum. It is this forum or nothing. The reason my heart thumps beforehand is because I fear we have the potential to do harm. However, I am also sure that someone who cannot sit through a fictionalized narrative in a lecture theatre will not be able to cope with dealing with their first death, or the first death where they know they omitted to do something, or the death of the first patient they have really built a relationship with. And they will not have the ability to opt out. Students can opt out of death and dying for the whole of their training, but not once they qualify. On her evaluation form a woman who was terribly distressed wrote 'Don't change anything. You have to do this'.

Evaluation of narrative and storytelling in education and training

The ultimate evaluation of any teaching about palliative care should be its impact on patient care, but since palliative care and medicine continue to struggle to evaluate the outcomes of palliative care clinical interventions, how teaching impacts on patient care is even more problematic. Very few palliative care education studies attempt to evaluate whether teaching alters practice, most focus instead on students' confidence or perceived competence in caring for patients following educational input.

How, then, should we judge the quality of teaching utilizing narrative and storytelling? In their study Davidhizar and Lonser asked students to evaluate the use of storytelling as a teaching technique through agreeing or disagreeing with qualitative statements. Students agreed that the approach made class more interesting and helped them recall and remember facts by making content more real. They felt that time spent with stories was not wasted and that professional students could learn concepts through stories (Davidhizar and Lonser, 2003).

In research we are familiar with the concepts of reliability, validity, and reproducibility as markers of quality, however, these indicators are consistent with a positivist paradigm inconsistent with narrative methods. Criteria used to make judgements about the quality of narrative and action research seem more applicable to narrative inquiry in education. Such criteria continue to be debated and will depend upon the nature and purpose of the narrative inquiry, however they might include the principles of historical continuity (how the story arose historically), of reflexivity (the transparency of the narrator's description and presumptions), of dialectics (has the story developed in dialogue with others and is it authentic?), of workability (is the story ethical, does it empower others and suggest workable practices?) and of evocativeness (Heikkinen et al. 2007). Narrative inquiry also 'aims . . . for verisimilitude, or . . . the appearance of truth or reality' (Polkinghorne, 1998: 176).

The quality of narrative and storytelling in education should thus be judged upon whether it is explicit why stories are being sought and used: do the stories invoked appear real and believable; are they of aesthetic merit; do listeners connect with and respond to them; are they analysed critically; do they encourage democratic participation, exploration, and learning (Guba and Lincoln, 1989; Reason and Bradbury, 2001)?

Conclusions

The current turn to narrative in health care can help students and professionals to retain or regain their compassion and humanity in caring for patients and each other. Narrative and storytelling are familiar in clinical practice in palliative care; we relish caring for patients in the context of their 'whole' stories, and even in helping patients 'restory' their current situations to maintain or regain hope. We need to extend this familiarity with story into our teaching, mindful of the requirement for quality, in an effort to enable our future health care colleagues to maintain and replenish their humanity in order to provide the best possible patient care.

References

Belling, C. (2006) Medicine and the silent oracle: an exercise in uncertainty. *Journal of Learning through the Arts*, **2**, Article 3 available at: http://repositories.cdlib.org/clta/lta/vol2/iss1/art3 (Accessed 5 August 2008).

Bolton, G. (1999) Stories at work: reflective writing for practitioners. *Lancet*, **354**, 243–45.

Boyd, E. M. and Fales, A. W. (1983) Reflective learning: the key to learning from experience. *Journal of Humanistic Psychology*, **23**, 99–117.

Bruner, J. (1991) The narrative construction of reality. *Critical Inquiry*, **18**, 1–21.

Carter, B. (2006) 'One expertise among many' – working appreciatively to make miracles instead of finding problems: using appreciative inquiry as a way of reframing research. *Journal of Research in Nursing*, **11**, 48–63.

Carter, B. (2007) Kicking Eeyore into touch: 'Living-strong', 'nursing-strong' and being appreciative and solution-focused. *Contemporary Nurse*, **23**, 181–88.

Charon, R. (2000a) Literature and medicine: origins and destinies. *Academic Medicine*, **75**, 23–27.

Charon, R. (2000b) Reading, writing, and doctoring: literature and medicine. *American Journal of the Medical Sciences*, **319**, 285–91.

Charon, R. (2004) Keynote address: narrative in medicine. *Narrative based medicine conference*. British Medical Association, London.

Coles, R. (1989) *The Call of Stories: Teaching and the Moral Imagination*. Houghton Mifflin, Boston.

Cooperrider, D. (1990) Positive image, positive action: the affirmative basis of organizing. In *Appreciative Management and Leadership: The Power of Positive Thought and Action in Organizations* (ed. S. Srivastva and D. Cooperrider). San Fransisco, Jossey Bass, pp. 91–125.

Coulehan, J. (2007) Written role models in professionalism education. *Medical Humanities*, **33**, 106–09.

DasGupta, S. (2003) Reading bodies, writing bodies: self-reflection and cultural criticism in a narrative medicine curriculum. *Literature in Medicine*, **22**, 241–56.

Davidhizar, R. and Lonser, G. (2003) Storytelling as a teaching technique. *Nurse Educator*, **28**, 217–21.

Elwyn, G. and Gwyn R. (1999) Stories we hear and stories we tell: analysing talk in clinical practice. *British Medical Journal*, **318**, 186–88.

Ellershaw, J. and Wilkinson, S. (2003) *Care of the dying: a pathway to excellence*. Oxford University Press, Oxford.

Evans, B. and Severtsen, B. (2001) Storytelling as cultural assessment. *Nursing and Healthcare Perspectives*, **22**, 180–83.

Gergen, K. J. (1999) Affect and organization in post-modern society. In *Appreciative Management and Leadership* (ed. S. Srivastva and D. L. Cooperrider). Williams Custom Publishing, Euclid, Ohio. pp. 153–74.

Greenhalgh, T. (1999) Narrative based medicine: narrative based medicine in an evidence based world. *British Medical Journal*, **318**, 323–25.

Greenhalgh, T. and Hurwitz, B. (1999) Narrative based medicine: why study narrative? *British Medical Journal*, **318**, 48–50.

Guba, E. G. and Lincoln, Y. S. (1989) *Fourth Generation Evaluation*. Sage, Newbury Park.

Guyatt, G. H., Haynes R. B., Jaeschke, R.Z., Cook, D. J., Green, L., Naylor, C. D., Wilson, M. C. and Richardson, W. S. (2000). Users' Guides to the Medical Literature: XXV. Evidence-based medicine: principles for applying the users' guides to patient care. *Journal of the American Medical Association*, **284**, 1290–96.

Hart, E. (1996) Action research as a professionalizing strategy: issues and dilemmas. *Journal of Advanced Nursing*, **23**, 454–61.

Heikkinen, H. L. T., Huttunen, R., and Syrjälä, L. (2007) *Educational Action Research*, **15**, 5–19.

Hockley, J. and Froggatt, K. (2006) The development of palliative care knowledge in care homes for older people: the place of action research. *Palliative Medicine*, **20**, 835–43.

Hunter, L. P. and Hunter, L. A. (2006) Storytelling as an educational strategy for midwifery students. *Journal of Midwifery and Womens' Health*, **51**, 273–78.

Hunter, K. M., Charon R., and Coulehan, J. L. (1995) The study of literature in medical education. *Academic Medicine*, **70**, 787–94.

Inui, T. S. (2003) *A Flag in the Wind: Educating for Professionalism in Medicine*. Association of American Medical Colleges, Washington DC.

Inui, T. S. and Frankel, R. M. (2006) Hello stranger: building a healing narrative that includes everyone. *Academic Medicine*, **81**, 415–18.

Kleinman, A. (1988) *The Illness Narratives: Suffering, Healing and the Human Condition*. Basic Books, New York.

Launer, J. (1999) Narrative based medicine: a narrative approach to mental health in general practice. *British Medical Journal*, **318**, 117–19.

Levett-Jones, T. L. (2007) Facilitating reflective practice and self-assessment of competence through the use of narratives. *Nurse Education in Practice*, **7**, 112–19.

Myers Schim, S. and Raspa, R. (2007) Crossing disciplinary boundaries in end-of-life education. *Journal of Professional Nursing*, **23**, 201–07.

Polkinghorne, D. (1998) *Narrative knowing and the human sciences*. State University of New York Press, Albany.

Reason, P. and Bradbury, H. (2001) *Handbook of action research*. Sage, London.

Schön, D. (1983) *The Reflective Practitioner: How Professionals Think in Action*. Basic Books, New York.

Schwartz, M. and Abbott, A. (2007) Storytelling: a clinical application for undergraduate nursing students. *Nurse Education in Practice*, **7**, 181–86.

Schneider, B. and Caswell, D. (2003) Using narrative to build community and create knowledge in the interdisciplinary classroom. *History of Intellectual Culture*, **3**(1). Available at: http://www.ucalgary.ca/hic/issues/vol3/4 (Accessed 10 July 2008).

Sierpina, V. S., Kreitzer, M. J., MacKenzie, E., and Sierpina, M. (2007) Regaining our humanity through story. *Explore (NY)*, **3**, 626–32.

Taylor, B., Bulmer, B., Hill, L., Luxford, C., Macfarlane, J. and Stirling. K. (2002) Exploring idealism in palliative nursing care through reflective practice and action research. *International Journal of Palliative Nursing*, **8**, 324–30.

Wright, M. and Baker, A. (2005) The effects of appreciative inquiry interviews on staff in the UK National Health Service. *International Journal of Healthcare Quality Assurance*, **18**, 41–61.

Chapter 8

Patient and carer narratives and stories

Phil Cotterell, Helen Findlay, and
Ann Macfarlane MBE

Within this chapter we are concerned with the role and use of patient and carer stories as a part of 'user involvement' initiatives in palliative care. We propose that experiences, which may be presented as narrative or storied accounts, are a form of knowledge that can and should be utilized to greater effect in palliative care. Rather than perceiving stories as passive – albeit perhaps interesting accounts – we propose that narratives and stories can have positive personal impacts upon the authors and, importantly, on palliative care practitioners and organizations. We will argue that the transformation of professional practice and services through an engagement with the stories of palliative care service users needs to be done in a way where narratives and stories are not just viewed as complaints to be handled individually (not all of them will necessarily highlight problems; some may describe good practice that could be disseminated to others). Rather, we believe they should be seen collectively, and with regard to the specific organizational structures and cultures of services, as well as in terms of the wider social context, so that stories are turned into issues.

Further in this chapter we present two storied accounts by Helen and Ann and reflect on the potential for learning that may be possible in palliative care if such stories were attended to more effectively. First, we present an introduction to service user involvement and consider the connections with narratives and stories.

Service user involvement

There has been a changing relationship in recent years between those of us who need to make use of health and social care services and those who provide them. The relationship has been moving away from one based on paternalism towards a more equal relationship in which those people in receipt of services have a greater say with regard to how they are provided and care is delivered (Davies et al. 2006: 28). This new relationship, in which conventional understandings of professional and patient is refashioned, has simultaneously been referred to as service user involvement, patient and public involvement, or more generally as participation or partnership working.

The language of involvement is wide-ranging, confusing, and at times seemingly contradictory. It is important to be clear at the outset of what we mean by the terms we use in this chapter. We have chosen to use the term 'service user' to describe those people who make use of health and social care services (including carers and family members); and 'service user involvement' to describe processes where the views and priorities of service users inform the delivery of services. While we are aware that the term 'service user' can be contentious and disliked by some people, a passive and restrictive interpretation is not intended here and we recognize that being a service user is but one aspect of a person's life.

The rationale for ensuring that service users are at the centre of practice, policy and research in health and social care is fundamentally about learning from direct first-hand experience that service users, rather than professionals, have gained. It is anticipated that such learning will lead to improvements in the way services are provided, and will make them more responsive to the needs of those they are intended to support. At a minimum then, service user involvement is about making services and the way they are provided, better for those who require them now and also in the future. And at the heart of service user involvement is a concern about practice and with the nature of relationships between those who provide and those who use services.

Through legislation and policy directives, service user involvement has become a central component of health and social care provision in the United Kingdom (Department of Health, 1999; 2001; 2006). However, while there may well be a political drive for participation and public involvement in policy agenda, a so-called 'bottom up' drive from service users for greater inclusion and participation has also been identified (Beresford and Croft, 2001). Jenny Morris endorses this in noting the 'insistence by historically powerless groups that they want to be involved in decisions which determine the quality of their lives' and that they want 'their voices heard, to be part of their community rather than set apart from it' (Morris, 1994: 1).

There is a clear 'activist' element to challenges laid down by disabled people, for example, which led to a reconsideration of assumptions about disabled people and their place within society (see Campbell and Oliver, 1996). An important aspect of this activist or bottom-up commentary from service users was the challenge it raised to professional dominance, and the resistance it provided to professional – client relationships that can be dependency-creating (Oliver, 1990: 90). Service user involvement clearly has connections to the activism of disabled people over a considerable length of time. It is also grounded in the pressure from service users to reclaim their own experiences and knowledge (Beresford, 1999; 2003). In pursuit of this there has been awareness of, and emphasis on, the need to collectivize service user accounts in order to challenge policy and practice. There is a political and ethical imperative that acknowledges individual accounts, or stories, while striving to challenge and influence by way of pooling experience and knowledge.

Involvement in palliative care

Service user involvement has only relatively recently been developed within palliative care. This is perhaps surprising considering the underlying philosophy of the specialty that has promoted a partnership approach between service user, carers, and professionals (Faull, 1998: 3). Tenets of mutual respect, listening, and agreeing priorities and goals, have been central in this philosophy (Twycross, 1995: 4).

Cicely Saunders, a widely acknowledged leader in the development of the modern hospice and palliative care movement, intended the movement 'to be a voice for the voiceless', and to 'enable people who were facing the end of their lives . . . to speak to people outside' (Oliviere, 2000: 103). The importance of listening to and learning from service users was critical to Saunders, but her work can also be read as a more radical call for engagement, dialogue, and co-production with dying people and carers. Indeed, Cicely Saunders' relationship with David Tasma, a dying man she met in her role as a hospital almoner, was foundational in her ideas about hospice care (Du Boulay, 1984: 57). Saunders' version of dialogue, involved a ceding of professional authority to patients and carers, enabling alternative views and voices to emerge and to question and improve existing practices and care relationships.

Despite the apparent 'fit' between user involvement and palliative care philosophy, there has been a great deal of scepticism and caution regarding the development of service user involvement initiatives in palliative care practice and research (Gott, 2004; Payne, 2002; Small and Rhodes, 2000). It has been suggested that 'considerable paternalism' exists in palliative care (Randall and Downie, 2006: 20) which needs to be challenged as a part of user involvement. Consideration also needs to be given to the nature of involvement. To have an impact, whether at the level of improving practice and care relationships or at a policy level, involvement must be connected to change and improvement.

The development of the modern hospice movement in the United Kingdom can be seen to have developed from just such a desire to change and improve upon the existing provision of care and support for people affected by life-limiting conditions. It was also often the case that this impetus came from the use of personal experience, as for Saunders mentioned above. A large part of this development also stemmed from practitioners with an interest in palliative care, listening, learning, and responding to the 'voice of the patient' (Clark et al. 2005: 18). Indeed, it is important to recognize user involvement developments in palliative care (Beresford et al. 2000; Payne et al. 2005; Thomas, 2003) along with service user advocates (Broughton, 2003; Cotterell et al. 2007; Kraus et al. 2003; Paine, 2005).

Collectivizing stories

Both the individual and the collective 'voice' of service users have been important to the development of palliative care. Learning from the disabled people's movement and from organizations of service users, we can recognize the concern that individual voices are more likely to be marginalized. By collectivizing voice or first-hand accounts there is greater likelihood of real change ensuing (Branfield and Beresford et al. 2006: viii).

Within palliative care it may be that collectively bringing individual 'voices' together, perhaps by way of storytelling, is particularly important to reduce the effect of isolation and diminished impact. We will explore this point further in the last section. First, we will consider two storied accounts from service users that reflect on different experiences of palliative care.

Stories to challenge and improve palliative care

In this section we present two service user stories. Helen tells her family's story regarding the last days of their father's life, the issues that were raised during this period, and the action they took; and Ann relays her experience of accessing a hospice for symptom control.

Fighting motor neurone disease – Helen's story

Discovering that my elderly father had been left lying flat on his back in a wet, soiled, and very cold bed with red, running eyes, unable to hear as his hearing aid had come out and was somewhere in the bed, with a 'nil' by mouth message on the bed head, having lost his voice to the disease and breathing fitfully, was not the scene my brother had expected when visiting my father on his second day in an acute hospital.

My father had had Motor Neurone Disease (MND) diagnosed a few weeks before and, because he had become so malnourished, it was felt that a peg feed operation was needed. What my family didn't expect was that my father would be treated so appallingly by health professionals who we had expected would take the greatest care of him. I can forgive their lack of knowledge about MND as a rare condition – that ravages the body of the sufferer but leaves the mind as it is – but the seeming lack of compassion and humanity of some of them in dealing with him and us, was unforgiveable.

This experience, and unfortunately many others that my father had to endure from health services, in particular, and social care services in the community, care home and hospital over the seven weeks that he fought this disease from the time of diagnosis, were defining moments in strengthening the determination of us all (me as his youngest daughter, my two brothers, sister, and sister-in-law) to keep a record of everything that had occurred just before his diagnosis and during the course of his 'treatment.' We wanted to have something we could use in the future.

My father had cared for my mother over the last eight years of his life as she gradually declined into dementia and was herself in hospital during some of this period. If we hadn't been there to help them and try to make sense of the requirements of a health and social care system that seemed more concerned about process than outcome, then I hate to think what would have happened to them both.

So where were the palliative care services during all this? Precisely, the question we were asking. Where were they? Why was there no co-ordination between my father's hospital ward and the palliative care services? It was left to us to make the connection and to work out how to contact them.

After asking many questions on the ward, over a week after he had been admitted, a Macmillan palliative care nurse was pointed out to us just down the corridor. My sister flew down that corridor and virtually rugby-tackled the nurse and brought her to see my father. The nurse was very concerned about the condition of my father and that she hadn't been called to see him sooner.

The palliative care nurse organized an appointment as quickly as she could for an assessment of my father to be carried out by a palliative care consultant from the local hospice with a view to admitting him. This consultant visited my father a few days later which was the morning of the day that he died. It was all too late.

My father died a few minutes before 10:00 p.m. Just after 10:00 p.m. my family, the Macmillan nurse, and me were in the ward visitor's room and we began talking about what we would do next. In spite of the shock, numbness, and deep emotional upset that I felt, having been holding my father's hand just a few minutes earlier as he slipped away, I was determined to hold it together. I was determined that the health service would not be let off the hook and that I would go into battle if necessary on my father's behalf. We all believed they had let my father down very badly and had treated my family as though we were intruders to be patronized and not people who should be involved every step of the way.

But our actions weren't going to be in the form of a complaint that would probably get lost in bureaucracy forever and a day, and not help to actually make changes. We resolved to do something different and to present our concerns in a way that would be a more fitting legacy to my father's memory. 'The Findlay Report' was the result of our resolve (Findlay, 2006).

In the introduction to our Report, I wrote: 'this is the family's attempt to communicate constructively with the health and social services professionals who sought to deal with our father's condition – and who did so with varying degrees of usefulness, compassion and understanding. We only wish those same professionals had sought to communicate with us and between themselves in a similar manner' (Findlay, 2006: 3).

The main sections of the Report are a day-by-day diary of my father's experiences, covering a four-month period starting from just before his diagnosis and up to his death. There is also a section highlighting problems in communication and co-ordination within and between health and social services. In addition to identifying these issues as problems that should be addressed with health and social care professionals, we offered recommendations to help resolve the problems.

Once the Report was written and compiled, what to do with it? The way that it is written and the tone is important – it is deliberately inclusive. We did not want to alienate the individuals to whom we intended to send our report. We didn't pull any punches in the criticisms we had – we felt it important that these points were made – but by also offering possible solutions we hoped these would prompt those who received our Report to engage with us and possibly agree to meet and talk with us.

Drawing upon guerrilla tactics, we decided that in order to get maximum impact, we should target our Report at those individuals who we considered to be influential in the realm of decision and policy-making at local and national levels.

We already knew of many individuals at the local level in health and social services where my father lived so we initially sent our Report (either in hard copy form or via email) to those professionals. However, we also wanted to have influence on a wider scale as we believed our experience had broader implications and any lessons learnt could be applied to other parts of the United Kingdom. So we targeted individuals and organizations that we considered to have influence at a national level. For instance, individuals at the Department of Health responsible for drawing up and implementing health and social care policies, academics, government ministers and MPs, the Prime Minister, Healthcare Commission, Commission for Social Care Inspection, and the MND Association. Our Report has been going out to people on a regular basis over the two years since my father died. We have directly sent out around 80 copies so far and many of the recipients have been passing it on, so that well over 100 major players covering policy and practice in health and social services at local and national levels have seen its contents.

Reflecting on our story

Responses to our Report have been very positive. We were invited as a family to a number of meetings with the local hospital trust and Primary Care Trust (PCT) who were concerned to learn from our Report and to come up with some possible solutions that they could implement. Also, the senior nurse at the local Macmillan Unit who came to see my father when he was in hospital, gave us a lot of support when our Report first came out and identified useful people for us to send it to and gave copies to other people herself. She has also incorporated major parts of our report into training programmes that she supervises at the Unit to help their staff better understand what MND is and how to care for sufferers who are admitted to the Unit – an important activity as many Macmillan Units are now accepting MND patients, whereas only a couple of years or so ago they only accepted those with cancer.

Individuals from local health authorities have told us that they are also incorporating much of our Report in their own training courses. We have had positive responses from some major national players working in the realm of health and social care with a very senior official saying that he would use our Report to inform his future work. Some of those who responded also said that they have forwarded it to appropriate people in other parts of the United Kingdom. So we are hopeful that we are having an effect away from my father's local area and that is what we wanted.

We are still working with the hospital personnel where my father spent the last two weeks of his life – clinicians including neurologists, palliative care specialists plus social care professionals, representatives from the PCT, senior nurses, a regional representative from the MND Association, and others. We meet regularly with them as a part of a group, coordinated by a senior consultant. One of the reasons the consultant was able to establish this group was because of our Report, and through the group we have been able to talk about practical changes that can be made to their hospital processes to start to improve the problems that we had identified. There is a determination from all concerned that these meetings should not be 'talking shops' but should lead to practical changes. So we are part of a team that is trying to deliver an MND pathway that will cover the area where my father lived and beyond. Changes are happening on the ground and there is the will, following the details of my father's dreadful experience, to make necessary changes to turn the hospital into a centre of excellence for the treatment and care of people with MND and other neurological conditions. There is a way to go yet, but if this is achieved, then it would be a wonderful legacy to him.

Team Findlay

The Findlay Report was written from our notes and collective memories during the three months after my father's death. Writing was a difficult process at times for all the family. Thinking about my father's treatment, images of the way he looked because of the disease, and how he was treated, often flashed into my mind and caused great upset. But I was resolved to carry on. If he could show such courage in the face of this awful disease and the treatment he received than I could do this.

I didn't know how I would feel about talking to other people about our Report until I started attending meetings, along with my other siblings. But attending these meetings as a family meant that we provided our own support group – Team Findlay as I call it. We would get together before an appointment to talk about what we were going to say and who would say what. We tried to approach it as a business meeting and to get our points across, although emotions would bubble up every so often. I often felt like my insides were being serrated to hear myself talking about my father and what had happened, but I made myself immune to the pain at the time. We would then gather as a family after a meeting, to talk it through and decide what we were going to do next, and to offer solace to each other. I found that it was a day or two after a meeting that I would start to feel the pain both physically and emotionally – the anaesthetic that I had induced in myself to get me through it would wear off. It did start to get easier over time.

I believe that the emotional side of this kind of storytelling is an important element. I know there is the belief that in order to organize and run things properly and efficiently in the health services particularly, but also in social services, individuals have to set their emotions aside. But how can this possibly be appropriate when dealing with people who are in need of palliative and end-of-life care?

It's surely not beyond the wit of twenty-first century man and womankind to come up with a better and workable solution. For this to happen, it shouldn't be seen as the preserve of a few professionals to come up with the answers but rather as a concern for all of us – service users in particular.

The lived experience of hospice and palliative care – Ann's story

At the time of my referral to a hospice counsellor I was unable to predict that the experience would have such distinctive outcomes. I was referred because of deep emotional trauma caused by many years of hospitalization that began at the age of four. It took a long time for me to recognize that I required help, and, initially, I was referred to a psychologist entrenched in a medical model approach and from whom it took me 12 months to extricate myself. This person lacked awareness of disability issues, so that I was placed in the role of educator. He told me that he sat in sight of the door as he thought that if I got angry I might harm him with my wheelchair! I left sessions in a very difficult and often more negative place than on arrival.

The hospice counsellor came from a very different perspective that enabled me to explore the past in a way that shifted and moved part of a gigantic pile of rocks without any falling in on me. Soon after this referral, I was referred on to a hospice community palliative care team that specialized in pain management. This was another new experience, not all positive because most nurse practitioners were trained in a medical model. The positive aspect was that they had a great deal of time for me and tried hard to accommodate my independent approach to my long-term situation. It did, however, feel like a power struggle as I tried to maintain control while exercising choice.

A critical point came when the medication required for pain relief made me feel extremely ill and it was felt wise to admit me to the hospice for stabilization of the medication. In advance of admission, ward staff were informed that I was a very independent individual. This message was translated as 'leave her to manage, as she likes to do everything for herself'. From the moment of entering a side room, apart from specific medical input, I was left to my own devices. The medication made me feel over-anxious. Being left alone was a frightening experience and physically I was unable to manage anything on my own from a prone position in bed; I could not reach my light switch, call button, locker, water, or radio. I could not get up out of bed as I was unsure of the floor covering. Hospital environments are notorious for slippery floor surfaces and spillages and if a person uses crutches, sticks, or has mobility difficulties, their lives are put at risk on getting out of bed.

As soon as I began to recover from the negative effects of the medication I discharged myself. Staff showed anger, annoyance, and kept asking me why I should want to leave before I was fit enough. I, too, was angry and upset, and not in an emotionally secure place to explain my reasons for leaving the hospice. I was labelled a 'patient' rather than a 'person' and while

I saw the need to educate staff, I had no intention of taking on a teaching role. My professional life focused on the role of educator and at this time I was trying to sort out my personal life and I did not want the two to become confused. I desperately wanted some conversation, compassion, and to be understood and I left the hospice feeling completely at odds with the system and staff.

Writing about this period in my life has heightened my emotional state. I feel tension rising and ambivalence around the experience. On the one hand, I am indebted to the hospice for providing a counsellor who, to a great extent, freed me from the shackles that bound me to my childhood and teenage experiences, and my gratitude remains for her seven years of dedication. The years of input from the community palliative care team who assisted me in pain management enhanced my life and the medical effect of this treatment continues to the present time.

Reflecting on hospice and palliative care

Hospice and palliative care practices continue to operate mostly within a medical model. This makes it a struggle for people with life-limiting conditions who may be desperate to experience a service that liberates rather than restricts their lives. I am a member of a national user group comprising people who use, have used, and who would like to access palliative care services. Some members have long-term or life-limiting conditions apart from those related to cancer. Group members focus on issues related to palliative care at national and local levels in the hope that a social model approach will permeate through the system and structures, enabling person-centred support. Only part of day-to-day living focuses on our medical condition/s and our lives are far greater than those conditions. Within a medical model an illness can feel all-consuming.

It is worth noting here, the difference between the medical and social models of disability. The traditional medical model of care places an onus and responsibility on individuals and on an individual's 'limitations' and 'impairments', whereas the social model of disability sees explanations of disability clearly lying with society itself. It focuses on 'disabling environments rather than individual impairments' (Campbell and Oliver, 1996: 20). The social model highlights that disabled people need to be accepted for who they are. Impairment cannot be changed. However, disabling environments, systems, and attitudes can be changed ensuring barrier-free, inclusive communities for all people.

For more than twenty years I have been working with professional practitioners in health and social care and with disabled people on issues that relate to empowerment. This work includes personal development and understanding legislation, policy and practice to ensure that service users get their needs met through a social model approach that provides positive outcomes. This work has often come at an enormous physical and emotional cost, but it is valuable if it results in service users experiencing choice and control, and lives worth living.

I am in a very different place when in the role of service user to that of my role as a disability rights and independent living consultant. When at events and meetings in my role as a service user I want other professional people to acknowledge that I am an expert by personal experience, and also that I bring more collective experience and knowledge of those who use services and to whom I have listened over many years. In this way I can share this experience and knowledge to shape policy and service provision. Not all disabled and ill people have this collective knowledge on which to draw but they are 'experts in their own individual experience' and this expertise should be valued and recognized.

Developing services and practice: storytelling in palliative care

In introducing this chapter we questioned whether narratives and stories could be utilized in palliative care as a mechanism for service improvement and/or practice development. Learning from developments in service user involvement, we acknowledged the possibility for service user experiences becoming part of an improvement agenda within palliative care.

We have seen from both Helen and Ann's storied accounts of palliative care that such accounts provide many learning opportunities for both palliative care practitioners and services. However, we are also aware of wider debates about the dangers of taking narratives and stories at face value and of the need to think critically about 'experience' (see Paley and Eva this volume). We are also aware that the narratives and stories of those who are socially marginalized are seldom heard. These issues raise fundamental questions and challenges about how palliative care services can learn from the accounts of service users in ways that promote critical dialogue and which recognize difference and diversity. And they raise questions for involved service users and involvement initiatives.

In engaging with these challenges we would suggest a complementary facet of 'narrative vigilance' (Paley and Eva, 2005), that alerts us to the differences that can exist between the emotional cadence of an account and external events. While recognizing the analytic value of these distinctions, we would argue that the emotionality of service user stories are both an integral part of the meaning of wider events and can also provide insight into more elusive aspects of the organizational culture and climate of palliative care services – how services and care 'feel'. It is vital therefore that dual attention is given to both 'how things have happened' *and* to 'how things feel' in interpreting the stories of service users (Paley and Eva, 2005) and in drawing out their implications for service development.

While there are significant differences between Helen and Ann's stories, it is also clear that both stories have a strong emotional element that leave the reader thinking that it could and should have been different for them. It has also been an emotional journey for them as well, and this 'emotional cost' should not be underestimated for any service user who offers or who is requested to 'tell their story'. The meanings that a storyteller conveys need to be believed, the implications taken seriously, and acted upon where appropriate.

There is a danger that the service users' experience will not be believed, or there may be a suggestion that the person is unrepresentative, or is purely seeking attention. The possibility for the veracity or integrity of the storyteller to be doubted has been acknowledged elsewhere (Eva and Paley, 2006). This assumption though is likely to be to the detriment of the persons' integrity and well-being and can have serious consequences. It is often only when people have experienced a similar situation and can identify with the storyteller that the story teller gains credibility and is believed.

Consideration also needs to be given to the timing of when service users are asked to provide stories and the fact that some service users may not want to dwell on their story needs to be acknowledged. For some, storytelling may be emotionally helpful in a variety of ways. However, for others it can also be distressing to recount negative experiences. This may be especially so for bereaved carers.

Another important and related aspect concerns ownership of stories. Once a story 'goes public' the experience is a shared story. It makes connections with others who may be interested, sympathetic, critical, or unconcerned. Perhaps also the storyteller joins with other storytellers who have had similar experiences and becomes part of a 'community of survivorship' (Frank, 2003). Storytelling, then, may at one level be seen as an individual act but at another as a social act, mediated by and responsive to others.

In acknowledging the role that stories told by people with mental health problems have had in challenging the dominant medical model in psychiatry, Barnes (2006: 31) indicates a political dimension to storytelling. Whether for people with mental health problems, or for disabled people, or for people with life-limiting conditions, relaying one's own experiences in the form of a story, video diary, blog, or a piece of art or drama, there can be a sense of making the hidden visible. This may be especially so where there are perceived injustices, unresponsive services, or unsatisfactory professional practice.

In a discussion of self-help/mutual-aid groups, it is highlighted how collective knowledge production gained via participation with people having similar experiences to oneself can also be seen as an informal political activity, that can be challenging and/or complementary to more formal political activities (Munn-Giddings, 1998: 91). There can be influences that filter wider than the group itself as well as internal group-related influences such as personal development, creativity, ownership, and empowerment (Munn-Giddings, 2001). Influencing and instigating change, however, is often far more difficult to achieve and a 'lone voice' may well find themselves in a poor bargaining position. There can also be a heightened sense of vulnerability in relaying individual accounts that are challenging to the service you are reliant upon. Harnessing individual stories and individual voices collectively may offer the impetus that palliative care organizations require to listen, act, and change in response to these stories:

> If we wish to promote the use and usefulness of user voices in palliative care we need to help systems of decision-making and of education change so that users are made more skilful at engaging with technical knowledge, and professionals are made more susceptible to embodied knowledge. We have to understand how bringing together users and a range of professionals creates an organizational structure that learns and changes together.
>
> (Small, 2005: 72)

Storytelling has the capacity to induce emotion in the reader, and perhaps, to appreciate the injustice or dissatisfaction raised by the storyteller. Learning from work in service user involvement we advocate that reaching an understanding of an experience is the first step. Following being challenged by the story and engaging with it, the next and very important step, is being moved to act because of it.

To act is vital. In order to facilitate the use of stories in service development thought needs to be given to practical methods that can be employed. Effective processes and structures need to be in place. Beyond effective processes for capturing collective storied accounts are outcomes. Having definable and properly evaluated outcomes is very important; otherwise how do we know whether the stories generated have any significant impact on policy and practice?

Stories, such as those presented in this chapter, can be powerful and have an important message to convey. Palliative care needs to view the stories raised by service users as a constructive 'critical perspective', and as an invitation to dialogue and action.

References

Barnes, M. (2006) *Caring and Social Justice*. Palgrave Macmillan, Basingstoke, UK.

Beresford, P. (2003) *It's Our Lives: A Short Theory of Knowledge, Distance and Experience*. OSP for Citizen Press, London, UK.

Beresford, P. and Croft, S. (2001) Service user's knowledges and the social construction of social work. *Journal of Social Work*, 1(3), 295–316.

Beresford, P., Broughton, F., Croft, S., Fouquet, S., Oliviere, D., and Rhodes, P. (2000) *Palliative Care: Developing User Involvement, Improving Quality*. Centre for Citizen Participation, London, UK.

Beresford, P. (1999) Making participation possible: movements of disabled people and psychiatric survivors. In *Storming the Millennium* (eds. T. Jordan and A. Lent). Lawrence and Wishart, London, UK. pp. 34–50.

Branfield, F. and Beresford, P. with Andrews, E. J., Chambers, P., Staddon, P., Wise, G., and Williams-Findlay, B. (2006) *Making User Involvement Work: Supporting Service User Networking and Knowledge*. Joseph Rountree Foundation, York, UK.

Broughton, F. (2003) Conclusion: Thoughts of a palliative care user. In *Patient Participation in Palliative Care: A Voice for the Voiceless* (eds. B. Monroe and D. Oliviere). Oxford University Press, Oxford, pp. 196–99.

Campbell, J. and Oliver, M. (1996) *Disability Politics: Understanding Our Past, Changing Our Future*. Routledge, London, UK.

Clark, D., Small, N., Wright, M., Winslow, M., and Hughes, N. (2005) *A Bit of Heaven for the Few: An Oral History of the Modern Hospice Movement in the United Kingdom*, Observatory Publications, Lancaster, UK.

Cotterell, P., Clarke, P., Cowdrey, D., Kapp, J., Paine, M., and Wynn, R. (2007) Becoming involved in research: a service user research advisory group. In *Creative Engagement in Palliative Care – New Perspectives on User Involvement* (ed. L. Jarrett). Radcliffe Publishing Ltd, Abingdon, UK. pp. 101–15.

Davies, C., Wetherell, M., and Barnett, E. (2006) *Citizens at the Centre: Deliberative Participation in Healthcare Decisions*. The Policy Press, Bristol, UK.

Department of Health (2006) *Our Health, Our Care, Our Say: A New Direction for Community Services*. DH, London, UK.

Department of Health (2001) *Health and Social Care Act 2001*. DH, London, UK.

Department of Health (1999) *Patient and Public Involvement in the New NHS*, DH, London, UK.

Du Boulay, S. (1984) *Cicely Saunders. The Founder of the Modern Hospice Movement*. Hodder and Stoughton, London, UK.

Eva, G. and Paley, J. (2006) Stories in palliative care. *Progress in Palliative Care*. 14(4), 155–64.

Faull, C. (1998) The history and principles of palliative care. In *Handbook of Palliative Care* (eds. C. Faull, Y. Carter and R. Woof). Blackwell Science Ltd, Oxford, UK. pp. 1–12

Findlay, H. (2006) *The Findlay Report: Case Study on the Handling of a Case of Motor Neurone Disease by Health and Social Care Services in the UK*. Unpublished report. Available from: findlay.helen@googlemail.com

Frank, A. W. (2003) Survivorship as craft and conviction: reflections on research in progress. *Qualitative Health Research*, 13(2), 247–55.

Gott, M. (2004) User involvement and palliative care: rhetoric or reality? In *Palliative Care Nursing: Principles and Evidence for Practice* (eds. S. Payne, J. Seymour and C. Ingleton). Open University Press, Maidenhead, UK. pp. 75–89.

Kraus, F., Levy, J., and Oliviere, D. (2003) Brief report on user involvement at St Christopher's Hospice. *Palliative Medicine*, **17**, 375–77.

Morris, J. (1994) *The Shape of Things to Come? User-led Social Services*. National Institute for Social Work, London, UK.

Munn-Giddings, C. (2001) Links between kropotkin's theory of 'mutual aid' and the values and practices of action research. *Educational Action Research*, **9**(1), 149–58.

Munn-Giddings, C. (1998) Self-help/mutual aid, gender and citizenship. In *Shifting Bonds, Shifting Bounds: Women, Mobility and Citizenship in Europe* (eds. V. Ferreira, T. Tavares and S. Portugal). Celta Editora, Oeiras, Portugal. pp. 85–94.

Oliver, M. (1990) *The Politics of Disablement*. The Macmillan Press Ltd, London, UK.

Oliviere, D. (2000) A voice for the voiceless. *European Journal of Palliative Care*, **7**(3), 102–05.

Paine, A. (2005) Users do not want to be treated with kid gloves. *Community Care*. 6–12 October, 33.

Paley, J. and Eva, G. (2005) Narrative vigilance: the analysis of stories in health care. *Nursing Philosophy*, **6**, 83–97.

Payne, S. (2002) Are we using the users? *International Journal of Palliative Nursing*, **8**(5), 212.

Payne, S., Gott, M., Small, N., Oliviere, D., Sargeant, A., and Young, E. (2005) *User Involvement in Palliative Care: A Scoping Study. Final Report to St. Christopher's Hospice*. June 2005, St. Christopher's Hospice, London, UK.

Randall, F. and Downie, R. S. (2006) *The Philosophy of Palliative Care: Critique and Reconstruction*, Oxford University Press, Oxford, UK.

Small, N. (2005) User voices in palliative care. In *Handbook of Palliative Care* (eds. C. Faull, Y. Carter and E. Daniels). 2nd edn, Blackwell, Oxford, pp. 61–73.

Small, N. and Rhodes, P. (2000) *Too Ill To Talk? User Involvement and Palliative Care*, Routledge, London, UK.

Thomas, J. (2003) *Care of the Dying and the NHS: Some Carers' Views*. The Nuffield Trust, London, UK.

Twycross, R. (1995) *Introducing Palliative Care*. Radcliffe Medical Press Ltd, Abingdon, UK.

Chapter 9

Mediator deathwork[1]

Tony Walter

A dead body tells no tales, except those which it
whispers to the quick ear of the scientific expert,
by him to be reported in the proper quarter.
Douglas Maclagan

'Forensic Medicine from a Scotch Point of View',
British Medical Journal, 17 August 1878: 237, cited in
Burney (2000: 107)

Most of the stories and narratives in this book are told by the living.
Dr Maclagan, however, suggests that the task of the pathologist (and one might
add, for the more distant dead, the task of the archaeologist) is to listen to what
the deceased, or rather their remains, have to say about how they lived and
died. A bereavement counsellor told me:

> When there's been some mystery about the death, or how it's happened, or you haven't
> had all your answers met about how or why, I wonder if you have to turn to someone
> else who has access to the beyond, to get some of those answers.

Some of this counsellor's clients, who were bereaved parents, took a great
interest in the autopsy (post-mortem) report, while others consulted spiritualist mediums – in every such case they had unanswered questions about
their child or its death. Both the pathologist and the medium 'has access to the
beyond' and can 'get some of those answers'.

Professional obituary writers also interrogate the dead, not directly in the
manner of the pathologist, the archaeologist, or (arguably) the spiritualist
medium, but they interrogate those who knew the dead and publish a story
about him or her. Funeral celebrants, increasingly popular in Australia,
New Zealand, and the United Kingdom, likewise interview the deceased's
associates and then construct, and at the funeral publicly perform, the
deceased's story. The western gunslinger knows that 'Dead men tell no tales',

but dead men and women do tell tales. They tell them in autopsies, in inquests, in spiritualist church meetings, and séances; and we tell their tales, often in public, in the register office, in obituaries, in funeral eulogies.

Although pathologists' reports and consultations with mediums are not always for public dissemination, often they are. The pathologist's report becomes part of the highly public coroner's inquest (which in turn may be reported in the local news media), the medium may provide a public reading in the context of a spiritualist church service, while the obituary and the funeral tribute are by definition public. Narratives about the dead are provided not just within the privacy of the family or within the privacy of professional relationships with patients and clients in palliative care, but some narratives, some full-blown stories (as in the funeral eulogy) are highly public (see Paley, and Eva this volume, for further discussion about the difference between narratives and stories).

How do mourners relate these public narratives to their own, private, narratives? Making sense of the deceased's life and death is a need felt by many mourners (Neimeyer, 2005). They may talk, to themselves and others, at length about the deceased's life (Walter, 1996), or recount over and over the details of the death. Bereavement counselling increasingly may include a degree of narrative therapy, in which the client works out a story about the deceased and what the deceased meant to them. The aim of such therapy is not to produce a story that is objectively correct about the past, but one that helps the client get through the present (Hoyt, 2000; Spence, 1982). How then does the mourner make sense of public/official narratives and incorporate them into their own story of the deceased's life and death? And how do those employed to produce these official or public narratives go about their, sometimes distinctly macabre, sometimes surprisingly life-enhancing, duty? In this chapter, I sketch the work of those professionals who produce these public narratives and stories, and discuss in whose interests they are working and what this can mean for mourners. Their work operates on very different principles from that of the counsellor-client or doctor-patient relationship.

The empirical basis of this chapter comprises observations of English spiritualist churches in the late 1990s and interviews with bereavement counsellors about their clients' use of mediums (Walter, 2007); participation in the early stages of a research project on how mourners experience inquests (Davis et al. 2002); and my own involvement over several years in the training of both clergy and civil funeral celebrants (Institute of Civil Funerals, 2008). I also draw on and develop Ariès' (1981) concept of 'familiarity' with the dying and the dead, and my own earlier analysis of the biographical work done by mourners (Walter, 1996).

My earlier work has been criticized (Howarth, 2007) for implying that the stories mourners weave about the dead are static. Of course, they need not be static: the identities we create for the dead in everyday conversation and in other arenas evolve over time, just as do the identities we create for the living. What the present chapter shows is that stories about the dead work best for mourners when they are shareable, and when the various parties can co-construct the same story, or at least compatible stories. What gives such stories solidity is not that they are static, but that they are socially validated and bolstered by the stories of others. When private and public stories conflict, there is usually trouble in store – not least because some public stories (such as the inquest verdict, the newspaper obituary, or the funeral tribute) cannot be changed.

A sketch of mediator deathwork

Mediators are people who are skilled in bridging the gap between two different parties or two different worlds. The gap between the living and the dead is huge in post-Protestant and largely secular societies such as Britain where there are no formal religious channels for communicating with the dead – unlike Catholic countries, and unlike Japan and much of Africa where ancestors are venerated (Smith, 1974). The work of the professionals who tell dead people's tales is best characterized as mediation, for these professionals carry messages from the dead, or about the dead, to the living. It is no coincidence that the words 'medium' (she who brings messages from 'the other side') and the mass 'media' (which bring news, often about the dead, to an audience) share the same root.

The contours of mediator deathwork are as follows. My examples are from funeral celebrants, pathologists, coroners, and those spiritualist mediums who perform in the context of spiritualist churches (though these last are not normally recognized as 'professionals', they illustrate my argument well). I offer this sketch as a sociological 'ideal type', not meaning ideal in the sense of desirable, but as capturing the essence of this kind of work.

1. In human societies contact with the dead is often feared and always regulated. Certain occupations and roles are reserved for this dangerous work, and those engaged in it may attract either status or stigma (Parry, 1994). The modern mediator has a familiarity with the dead, denied to and/or shunned by the rest of us (Ariès, 1981). The pathologist has a familiarity with corpses; the spiritualist has a familiarity with spirits; the funeral celebrant and obituary writer know how to glean information about the dead immediately after the death when others may not know how to speak.

2. The mediator is instructed to find out about the dead. The corpse awaits the pathologist's scalpel; the funeral celebrant or obituarist is commissioned to write about the dead; the medium opens herself to receiving messages from the other side. Whether they like it or not, the dead are about to be interrogated.

3. The mediator receives information about, or a message from, the dead. The pathologist finds an enlarged liver; the medium hears the name 'Ethel', and feels love; the funeral celebrant talks to family members and gathers information about the deceased's life.

4. The mediator then edits the information into the form expected of him/her. From the enlarged liver, along with information about the deceased's lifestyle, the pathologist diagnoses alcohol poisoning. The medium concludes that this is Ethel's continuing spirit on the other side and that she is sending love to those on the earth plane. The funeral celebrant writes a personal tribute, encapsulating the deceased's life and character.

5. So far, the mediators have been working in private – the celebrant interviewing the family, the pathologist conducting the autopsy, the medium silently communing with the other side – but must now (and in the spiritualist's case, in a matter of micro-seconds) turn themselves into stage performers. They must perform their edited story in a ritual setting: the pathologist is interrogated by the coroner in a public inquest, the celebrant must perform the tribute at the funeral, the medium must pass the message on to the congregation or to the sitter.

6. In each case, the public rite is potentially tricky. The pathologist's diagnosis may be challenged; the celebrant must perform a tribute recognizable by all those present at the funeral, including ex-spouses and workmates as well as family members; the medium's message may not be 'taken' by the sitter. In each case, the authority of the mediator is vulnerable, and/or mourners may be disturbed by truths they would rather not face.

7. The public rite is tricky not only for the professional mediator, but also for others present (Howarth, 1997). At the inquest after a road traffic accident, the little boy's family find themselves within touching distance of the driver whose car killed him; at the funeral, wife and mistress meet for the first time; in the spiritualist meeting, some in the congregation are sceptical. Inquests and funerals can be highly charged, so the professional mediator needs to be skilled emotionally as well as in the more cognitive area of marshalling and presenting evidence (Biddle, 2003; Hockey, 1993; Wertheimer, 2001).

8. After the public rite, members of the audience may go through the mediator's performed story informally with each other. Whereas for the mediator the case is now over, this is not so for mourners. If the coroner seeks closure in the form of a verdict as to the cause of death, mourners need information about the death 'in order to compose the last stage of the deceased's biography and to map that narrative onto their own continuing biographies' (Hallam et al. 1999: 95). For them, this is a continuing process. One counsellor I spoke to accompanied two parents to the inquest of their dead child so 'they could check out with me whether their memory was similar to mine of what was said and what was done'. Funeral tributes may give permission to mourners to continue talking about the deceased in more informal settings in the days and weeks to come (Walter, 1996). In the United Kingdom, after Humanist or civil funerals, the celebrant normally hands the family a written version of the tribute; some families have used this as a starting point to develop their own scrapbook of memories. On my first visit to a spiritualist church, I was accompanied by a friend who chose to take notes when I was picked out by the medium; afterwards, she gave me the notes so I could remember what the medium had said and we discussed it together. Mediums often tape record private sittings for the sitter to take away afterwards.

9. Finally, the focus in both the private gleaning of information and the public performance of the edited story is not the bereaved, but the deceased. As Davis et al. note of the inquest, 'The deceased is the focus of the proceedings, rather than being a shadowy figure in someone else's story.' (Davis et al. 2002: ix)

In sum, the process is one in which information flows from *the dead* → *the mediator* → *public rite*. This triadic relationship between the dead, the mediator, and a public performance is very different from the dyadic therapeutic relationship: *client* ↔ *therapist*, or the *doctor* ↔ *patient* or *nurse* ↔ *patient* relationship. (→ refers to a one-way flow of information, ↔ to a two-way flow.)

Often the flow of information in mediator deathwork has more than three stages. The public rite of the inquest may determine that the deceased committed suicide, but this is not the end of the information flow. The verdict is then reported in the local newspaper, which is then read locally, and the news filters down into the school playground where the story is retold and the deceased's 7-year-old boy learns the news that shatters the story his mum told him of how his dad died. Private narratives that make comfortable sense of the death may have to come to terms with uncomfortable official narratives. And when there is an official cover-up, private narratives may have to come to terms with official narratives that the mourner knows to be incorrect, yet uncorrectable.

A mere channel?

Apart from wills, suicide notes and other deliberate communications – such as letters and videos – that dying people produce for mourners to read after the death, the information flows that mediator deathworkers deal in are not communicative acts, in that the dead do not initiate them. Rather, reading a cadaver, reading or hearing material produced by the deceased's intimates and associates, and possibly reading a spirit, is like reading any text: there is co-creation of meaning between the individual reader, his or her professional training, and text. Pathologists have been taught to read cadavers in certain ways, funeral celebrants have been taught to hear and edit mourners' stories in particular ways, professional obituarists know what to include and what to omit to make a readable story. This differs from counselling or curative medicine in that the text is the dead, not the living. Mediator deathworkers interrogate the dead, as literary critics interrogate a text.

Mediator deathworkers are required to underplay their own editorial work in telling the dead man's tale. When we look in detail at what makes a good medium, funeral celebrant, or pathologist, we find that they all are taught to be passive receptors of information. To quote a leaflet from the Spiritualists National Union (undated): 'The medium enters into the trance state, where their thoughts and personality are disengaged, so that the thoughts and personality of the communicator can be brought forward with as little interference as possible from the mind of the medium'. Exactly the same is true of funeral celebrants. In the training of funeral celebrants in which I have participated, some very talented trainees have failed the course because they could not keep themselves out of the picture. Their ego enabled them to be brilliant stage performers, but they could not resist inserting little bits of themselves into a picture that should be entirely about the deceased. At this point, we may note that in British newspapers such as the *Times* and *Daily Telegraph*, obituaries are the only major articles not signed by their author: the focus must be entirely on the deceased so that the writer becomes invisible. This is even true of pathologists. Whereas a medical diagnosis of the living often entails uncertainty, and different doctors may disagree on or debate the diagnosis, the autopsy is seen as the final court of appeal, in which the cadaver reveals the body's secrets. There is something final and definitive about the narratives performed by mediator deathworkers. If the process of narrative construction becomes apparent, its authenticity collapses.

In his book, *The Denial of Death*, Becker (1973) writes of how shamans, and Jesus, go to the land of the dead and return, thus becoming the divine heroes of traditional religions; soldiers who face death also return as heroes.

But spiritualist mediums, pathologists, funeral celebrants, and coroners neither are seen, nor portray themselves, as heroes. The reason, I suggest, is simple. Unlike Jesus they do not actually die; unlike shamans, they do not go through great physical trials and tribulations; unlike soldiers, they do not risk death. They visit the dead the easy way, at no risk to themselves. All they need is more or less training. So, their intimacy with the dead may be valued, it may be respected, but it is not heroic. These are modest men and women, who do modest work, and the narratives they recount about the dead are modest: his liver was enlarged, Doris sends her love, Fred was a decent husband. Unlike Jesus, and unlike New Age channellers (Spencer, 2001), these mediators do not return with myths or with a philosophy that might change the world. Rather, they return with mundane messages that help the living to get through the loss of one of their own by affirming their biographies of self and other, or by revising them, just a little bit; or in the case of pathologists, coroners, and registrars, their narratives enable the state to do its mundane work of compiling mortality statistics (Prior and Bloor, 1992).

Breaking bad news

So far, I have concentrated on autopsies, inquests, funerals, and spiritualist meetings. But there are several other settings in which the dead speak to the living, or in which information about the dead is ritually transmitted, performed, even paraded. These display some of the features of mediator deathwork.

One such group of settings concerns notification of the death. Sudnow (1967) has documented how hospital medical staff pass on bad news to relatives. The doctor must ascertain, from signs in and on the body, that it is, in fact, dead: *corpse → doctor → relatives*. Charmaz (1975) analyses how coroners' deputies in the United States pass on this information to relatives in cases where the relatives are unaware that the person is sick, let alone dead. Whereas the relative typically wants information about the death, the deputy has other concerns: to ensure that the family takes responsibility for disposing the body, and also to ensure that there is a neighbour or friend present to support the relative, so that the deputy can leave the house and get on with other cases.

Key family members then have the task of passing on news of the death to other family, and maybe friends and neighbours: *corpse → doctor → police officer/coroner's deputy → family → relatives, friends, neighbours*. The family are likely to insert a notice of the death and the funeral in the local newspaper, though the funeral director may do this for them. Death notices, as with other death mediations, are highly stylized, with particularly strong conventions as to wording: *corpse → doctor → family → funeral director → newspaper → readership* (O'Donohue and Turley, 2006).

In the United Kingdom, a close family member usually has to visit the local register office to register the death. Though the registrar's ten or so questions could be answered in just a few minutes, they often take half-an-hour, with the registrar prepared to act as sympathetic listener to the narrative of the death. Many informants recount the details of the actual death time and again, as though they need to get the facts straight, to get the narrative right, for their own as well as for others' benefits. Being legally required to recount the basic facts of the death to the registrar may therefore prompt a more extended narrative: *corpse → doctor → informant → registrar → public record.*

Other kinds of deathwork

Mediation is not the only kind of deathwork. There are, I suggest, several other types.

Barrier deathwork is well illustrated by the British funeral director. As in the United States the British corpse is removed to the funeral parlour, but there the similarity ends. Whereas the American funeral director transforms the corpse so that the wider community may commune with it in a public viewing, the British funeral director's main job is to look after the corpse, out of public view (Harper, 2007; Howarth, 1996). If any mourners come to view, it is in private, and alone or in groups of just two or three. If the corpse is disfigured, mourners may be actively discouraged from viewing. Children may be discouraged from viewing even good-looking corpses. The British funeral director's role is to protect the community at large from the dead, to assure the family that the body is being looked after by those who know about such things. The British funeral director's task is to keep the corpse within the private world of the family and close friends, thereby keeping the wider community of the living unfamiliar with the community of the dead, maintaining the barrier between the two.

Another, more partial, example of barrier deathwork concerns the suicide note. In the United Kingdom, suicide notes are the legal property of those to whom they are addressed, but between death and the inquest are legally appropriated by the coroner. There are cases where a coroner has chosen not to return the note, believing it would cause the family further distress; the family in turn do not know their legal right to ask for it back (Wertheimer, 1991: 77). Other examples of barrier deathwork are nurses who pull the curtains around the deceased's bed, and hospital porters who remove the corpse on a trolley designed to hide its true purpose. A number of sociological studies have studied barrier deathwork (Hockey, 1990; Howarth, 1996; Sudnow, 1967), and notions such as death denial (Kellehear, 1984), the sequestration of death (Mellor and Shilling, 1993), death as taboo (Walter, 1991), and hidden, forbidden or unfamiliar death (Ariès, 1981), all refer to professional deathworkers who hide death and the dead from laypeople.

Intercessory deathwork resembles mediator deathwork, except that the information flow is not from the dead to the living, but from the living to the dead. This is the essential work of the priest in religions such as Roman Catholicism in which prayers may be said for the dead. The mourner tells the priest of the person's death, and the priest prays to the saints (the sacred dead), who pray to God for the salvation of the deceased's soul: *mourner → priest → saints → God → soul.* Of course, this simplifies. In the complex and varied world of Catholicism, the information flow may be two way, with mourners looking for a sign from God or from the saints that all is well with the deceased.

Then there is *counselling deathwork*. Psychodynamic counselling neither crosses the barrier between the living and the dead, nor does it help create the barrier, it simply assumes it. In textbooks inclined to this view (e.g. Lendrum and Syme, 1992), and according to one anthropologist who observed workers in Cruse, Britain's largest bereavement counselling agency (Hockey, 1986), bereavement counsellors relate only to the living client; they see it as none of their business to relate to the dead, nor to look after the dead. Whatever the client says about the dead is translated by the counsellor into a story about the client's feelings (Walter, 1996: 17–19). The essential relationship is: *therapist ↔ client,* with the dead looking on, if at all, as mere bystanders.

Person-centred counsellors, however, are more likely to listen to their clients, unencumbered by particular theories of grief. One such counsellor (McLaren, 1998) sees herself as a 'companion and witness' to her client's experience, including any ongoing relationship with the deceased. She *is* concerned about the dead, her counselling role including helping clients to review their experience of the deceased and facilitating an evolving role for the deceased in their lives. Her experience echoes Klass' finding (1997) in a bereaved parents' group that their dead children gain a presence there that is difficult to achieve in other settings. Now that both bereavement research and teaching give more prominence to continuing bonds between mourners and mourned (Klass et al. 1996), counselling that takes these bonds seriously is gaining legitimacy. In Hedtke and Winslade's (2004) narrative approach to grief therapy, for example, the therapist actively facilitates the ongoing membership of the dead in a network of living relationships. Such therapists are not, however, mediators in my sense of gleaning information from the dead and passing it on, in public ritual, to the living, nor are they formally contracted – as are pathologists, coroners, mediums, obituarists, and funeral celebrants – to find out about the dead. Rather, they are engaged in *witnessing deathwork*, in which the deathworker is a witness to the mourner's entire experience, including any relationship with the one mourned. The relationship is *witness: mourner ↔ mourned.*

Skills

The skills and values required of counsellors and therapists are appropriate for their particular dyadic relationship with the client. 'Active listening', 'empathy', 'unconditional positive regard', and 'confidentiality' are the norms by which the therapist relates to the client. Such norms are relevant to mediator deathworkers insofar as they have to relate to mourners, but they are peripheral to the main task, namely relating to a dead body, a dead person, or a dead spirit. A funeral celebrant who listens actively to the feelings of the surviving members of the family, but does not get to the heart of what made the deceased tick, is not going to produce a good funeral. An obituarist who is empathetic but gets his facts wrong may lose his job. So, what values and skills do mediators between the dead and the living require?

First, they do need to show unconditional positive regard – to the dead. Showing respect to the dead is at the heart of mediator deathwork. The pathology professor instructs his students that, however indigent and drug-addicted the deceased may have been, throughout the autopsy they are to treat the corpse with respect (Fox, 1979). Funeral celebrants need to take such an interest in the deceased that they get to feel they actually knew them. At the end of an inquest or funeral, mourners will know that this death was taken seriously by the coroner or celebrant – a symbol that society takes this death, takes any death, seriously (Walter, 1990). If there is active listening, it is to the dead more than to the living; this is perhaps part of what people mean by paying respect, giving dignity, to the dead. Mourners and indeed society – through its coroners, registrars, and other mediators – pay respect to how each member of society lived and how they died.

Second, mediators need to be competent in gathering information, marshalling evidence, drawing conclusions from that evidence (e.g. about the cause of death, or the deceased's character), and presenting it. This ability to marshal evidence and draw conclusions is more akin to what scientists and lawyers do than to what narrative therapists do. Unlike narrative therapists, mediator deathworkers seek to construct a narrative that all those present can recognize; that can go on the public record; and that can stand the test of time. (These three aims can be contradictory, which is why the narrative does not always satisfy all parties and the occasion can be stressful.) It is the story's very public authority that may be helpful for mourners in validating the deceased's life and death – or unhelpful if they cannot integrate it into their own more subjective, private stories.

Mediator deathwork is therefore primarily rational, cognitive labour rather than emotional labour (Hochschild, 1983; James, 1992) – though death mediators also need to do emotional labour when in the presence of mourners. That said, holding the emotions of a diverse crowd of mourners needs more the skills of the actor than of the therapist. In my observation, funeral celebrants – who are paid by the chief mourner – actively engage in emotional labour, as indeed do clergy when they conduct funerals (Hockey, 1993). In contrast, British obituarists, like most professional journalists, are not routinely concerned about the emotional effect of their writing on families – they write not for the family, but for the newspaper's overall readership. By contrast, American and Australian lay obituarists writing in a local newspaper are performing emotional and/or narrative labour for a local readership comprising the deceased's mourners (Starck, 2006). The position of coroners, as we will see shortly, is more complex.

Third, mediators need to be able to perform on a stage, to project their voice, to hold an audience, while keeping their own personality out of the perform-ance. Of the two full-time marriage and funeral celebrants I interviewed during a visit to Australia in 1987, one had previously been his town's mayor, the other a journalist; each knew how to produce and edit a story to a deadline, and to perform it on stage.

None of these skills are core to counselling/therapy, indicating how different mediator deathwork is from counselling deathwork. This is not to say that a public telling of the dead (wo)man's tale may not be therapeutic for mourners. It will be therapeutic only if therapy is a side effect rather than the aim, and if two conditions are met that are very different from the therapeutic encounter: that the focus be on the deceased, and that the narrative be public and/or official.

In whose interests?

Mediator deathworkers vary in who they are working for. In England, pathol-ogists (when conducting coroner's post-mortems), coroners and registrars are commissioned by the state to find and record the deceased's identity and the time, place and cause of death. Their job is essentially legal/medical/bureaucratic. They are not paid to help the bereaved family. That said, many of them go beyond their core duty and go out of their way to provide information to the family with sensitivity, and choose not to air in public some of the harsher details of the case (Davis et al. 2002). Much of the emotional labour is done before the inquest, not by the coroner but by the coroner's officer or police family liaison officer, who work one-to-one with mourners and witnesses.

Other coroners, though, can be perceived as unfeeling. Families can be upset by a coroner who speaks in legal jargon or who mumbles, leaving them less rather than more clear as to why the person died. The Alder Hey (Royal Liverpool Children's Inquiry, 2001) and related scandals, in which pathologists retrained children's organs without gaining parental consent, led to distress among thousands of British parents. Newspaper reporting of inquests does not always spare the family's feelings.

It is debatable whether pathologists and coroners should be required to take account of the family's as well as the state's interest in gaining information about the death. There is merit in this argument, but it can be abused. I think of an inquest in which the coroner gave a verdict of accidental death to protect the family, but the train driver left the court confused and was unable to create any sense out of his trauma: he knew a suicide when he saw one. Maybe the coroner helped the family's grief, certainly he helped their standing in the local community, but he did not help the train driver's trauma.

The funeral celebrant is commissioned and paid by the family. But s/he has to produce a story that works not just for them but also for friends, colleagues, and neighbours. Different family members may have different perceptions of the deceased. Some may idealize the deceased; others may be glad s/he's gone. Yet everyone in the funeral has to recognize the picture painted. Not an easy task, which is why funeral celebrants receive considerable thanks when they get it right. One merit of the traditional Christian funeral, concerned to pronounce forgiveness of sin rather than to celebrate a life lived, is that no such definitive picture need be painted. Each mourner can read what they individually like into 'Forgive us our sins, as we forgive those who sin against us.' For better or for worse, talk of sin and worms has largely gone, even from Christian funerals, and celebration is what many now want. And celebration requires a story, not about Christ but about the deceased (Garces-Foley and Holcomb, 2005). Many clergy struggle to place the deceased's story within the larger Christian story (Quartier, 2007).

In New Zealand, where funeral celebrancy has a longer history as a profession than in the United Kingdom, celebrants are often not expected to produce one coherent eulogy, but to facilitate a range of family members and friends in telling their own stories about the deceased, and often there is no problem if the stories paint different pictures; mourners apparently do not demand consistency in the story (Shafer, 2007).

Conclusion

Over some decades, the characteristics of the dyadic *therapist ↔ client* relationship have been thoroughly explored, and it has become the ideological frame through which all forms of deathwork are seen. This may derive, in part, from the high status of the medical and psychological sciences (Rieff, 1966; Rose, 1989). Since the 1990s in the United Kingdom and perhaps elsewhere, the profile of bereaved people and their emotional needs has been rising rapidly, and there has been increasing pressure on a range of deathworkers – not least coroners and pathologists – to be more aware of mourners' emotional needs and to be trained accordingly. The triadic relationships of mediator deathwork, however, have yet to be explored. One implication is that, just as doctors are taught about the doctor–patient relationship and therapists about the therapist–client relationship, so funeral celebrants, coroners, and others should be taught about mediator deathwork. Training in narrative and storytelling should begin with those whose job it already is to produce public and/or on-the-record narratives about the dead!

One of the things that mourners may do is search for a story about the deceased's life and death that makes sense to them and that, ideally, can be shared with others (Neimeyer, 2001; Walter, 1996). The public narrating of the definitive story of that life and/or death – whether in inquest, funeral, or obituary – can be a key part of this process. If the public, publicized, narrative is acceptable, then this validates the deceased's life and its meaning to the mourner. But if the public narrative is unacceptable, incorrect, or misleading, then mourning becomes complicated by the drive to set the public record straight, or is compounded by extra grief over a last public statement that cannot now be corrected. For many people, the funeral tribute is the *only* occasion at which their story is publicly told, which perhaps is why professional funeral celebrants receive many letters of appreciation and have exceptionally high job satisfaction. Conversely, it is an indictment of the tribute-giver if mourners feel s/he failed to capture the essence of the person – as is often the case with British clergy, who are not trained to construct personal tributes and indeed may be theologically wary of them, yet are increasingly expected to produce such tributes. The only official account of the death occurs in registration and inquests; again, it is important that relatives can recognize the account told to registrars and by coroners. Putting on the public record a narrative that conflicts with the more comforting stories sometimes told by mourners is challenging work. Telling the dead (wo)man's tale – whether in funeral, obituary, registration, inquest, or séance – is a particular kind of work that needs to be understood, and valued, in its own right. For their part, mourners must marry their own private narratives with these more public narratives – and the marriage is not always easy.

Notes

1. This chapter is abridged from Tony Walter's (2005) Mediator deathwork. *Death Studies*, *29*(5), 383–412, Taylor and Francis, reprinted by permission of the publisher (Taylor and Francis Ltd., http://www.tandf.co.uk/journals). I acknowledge subsequent comments on that article by Kathryn Edwards, Ann Malamah-Thomas, Colin Murray Parkes, and Nigel Starck.

References

Ariès, P. (1981) *The Hour of our Death*. Allen Lane, London.

Becker, E. (1973) *The Denial of Death*. Free Press, New York.

Biddle, L. (2003) Public hazards or private tragedies? An exploratory study of the effect of coroners procedures on those bereaved by suicide. *Social Science and Medicine*, **56**, 1033–45.

Burney, I. (2000) *Bodies of Evidence: Medicine and the Politics of the English Inquest 1830–1926*. Johns Hopkins University Press, Baltimore.

Charmaz, K. (1975) The coroner's strategies for announcing death. *Urban Life*, **4**, 296–316.

Davis, G., Lindsey, R., Seabourne, G., and Griffiths-Baker, J. (2002) *Experiencing Inquests*. Home Office Research Study 241, London.

Fox, R. (1979) The autopsy: its place in the attitude-learning of second-year medical students. In *Essays in Medical Sociology, Journeys into the Field* (ed. R. Fox), pp. 51–77. Wiley, New York.

Garces-Foley, K. and Holcomb, J. S. (2005) Contemporary American funerals: personalizing tradition. In *Death and Religion in a Changing World* (ed. K. Garces-Foley and M. E. Sharpe). Armonk, NY.

Hallam, E., Hockey, J., and Howarth, G. (1999) *Beyond the Body: Death and Social Identity*. Routledge, London.

Harper, S. (2007) *Looking Death in the Face: A Comparative Ethnography of English and American Funeral Homes*. Paper given at the 8th International Conference on Death, Dying and Disposal, Bath.

Hedtke, L. and Winslade, J. (2004) *Re-membering Lives*. Amityville, Baywood NY.

Hochschild, A. (1983) *The Managed Heart*. Berkeley, University of California Press.

Hockey, J. (1986) *The Human Encounter with Death*. Durham University, unpublished PhD thesis.

_____ (1990) *Experiences of Death*. Edinburgh University Press, Edinburgh.

_____ (1993) The acceptable face of human grieving? The clergy's role in managing emotional expression during funerals. In *The Sociology of Death* (ed. D. Clark). Blackwell, Oxford.

Howarth, G. (1996) *Last Rites, The Work of the Modern Funeral Director*. Amityville, Baywood.

_____ (1997) Death on the road: the role of the English coroners court in the social construction of an accident. In *The Aftermath of Road Accidents* (ed. M. Mitchell). Routledge, London and New York.

Howarth, G. (2007) *Death and Dying: A Sociological Introduction*. Polity, Cambridge.

Hoyt, M. (2000) *Some Stories Are Better Than Others: Doing What Works in Brief Therapy and Managed Care*. Brunner/Mazel, New York.

Institute of Civil Funerals (2008) Available at: http://www.iocf.org.uk/.

James, N. (1992) Care = organization + physical labour + emotional labour. *Sociology of Health and Illness*, **14**(4), 488–509.

Kellehear, A. (1984) Are we a death-denying society? A sociological review. *Social Science and Medicine*, **18**, 713–23.

Klass, D. (1997) The deceased child in the psychic and social worlds of bereaved parents during the resolution of grief. *Death Studies*, **21**, 147–75.

Klass, D., Silverman, P. R., and Nickman, S. L. (eds) (1996) *Continuing Bonds, New Understandings of Grief*. Taylor and Francis, Bristol, PA and London.

Lendrum, S. and Syme, G. (1992) *The Gift of Tears*. Routledge, London.

McLaren, J. (1998) A new model of grief: a counsellor's perspective. *Mortality*, **3**, 275–90.

Mellor, P. and Shilling, C. (1993) Modernity, self-identity and the sequestration of death. *Sociology*, **27**, 411–32.

Neimeyer, R. (ed.) (2001) *Meaning Reconstruction and the Experience of Loss*. American Psychological Association Press, Washington, DC.

Neimeyer R. (2005) Grief, loss, and the quest for meaning. *Bereavement Care*, **24**(2), 27–30.

O'Donohue, S. and Turley, D. (2006), Service providers and bereaved consumers. *Human Relations*, **59**, 1429–48.

Parry, J. (1994) *Death in Banaras*. Cambridge University Press, Cambridge.

Prior, L. and Bloor, M. (1992) Why people die: social representations of death and its causes. *Science as Culture*, **3**, 346–64.

Quartier, T. (2007) *Bridging the Gaps: An Empirical Study of Catholic Funeral Rites*. Transaction, NY.

Rieff, P. (1966) *The Triumph of the Therapeutic: Uses of Faith after Freud*. Chatto, London and Windus.

Rose, N. (1989) *Governing the Soul: The Shaping of the Private Self*. Routledge, London.

Royal Liverpool Children's Inquiry (2001) *Royal Liverpool Children's Inquiry: Report*. London, House of Commons Available at: http://www.rlcinquiry.org.uk/.

Shafer, C. (2007) *Contested Tributes, Continuing Bonds and Living Memorials at Life-centred Funerals*. Paper given at the 8th International Conference on Death, Dying and Disposal, Bath.

Smith, R. J. (1974) *Ancestor Worship in Contemporary Japan*. Stanford University Press, Stanford.

Spence, D. P. (1982) *Narrative Truth and Historical Truth: Meaning and Interpretation in Psychoanalysis*. Norton, New York.

Spencer, W. (2001) To absent friends: spiritualist mediumship and New Age channelling compared and contrasted. *Journal of Contemporary Religion*, **16**, 343–60.

Spiritualists National Union (undated) *Leaflet no. 6, Phenomena*. Stanstead, Spiritualists National Union.

Starck, N. (2006) *Life After Death: The Art of the Obituary*. Melbourne University Publishing, Melbourne.

Sudnow, D. (1967) *Passing On: The Social Organization of Dying*. Englewood Cliffs, Prentice Hall.

Walter, T. (1990) *Funerals: And How to Improve Them*. Hodder, London.

____ (1991) Modern death: taboo or not taboo? *Sociology*, **25**, 293–310.

____ (1996) A new model of grief, bereavement and biography. *Mortality*, **1**, 7–25.

____ (2007) Mediums and Mourners. *Theology*, **110**(854), 92–100.

Wertheimer, A. (1991) *A Special Scar: The Experiences of People Bereaved by Suicide*. Routledge, London.

Section 3

Working with patients and carers

Chapter 10

The necessity and dangers of illness narratives, especially at the end of life

Arthur W. Frank

At the core of the practice of care is storytelling. Philosophers (MacIntyre, 1984), neuroscientists (Damasio, 2000; 2003), and anthropologists (Cruikshank, 1998) all agree that human beings are storytelling creatures, conditioned by our collective history and possibly hardwired in our bodies not only to report our experiences and emotions in story, but to *discover* who we are through telling stories. To attend to a person's stories is to enable his or her self-discovery, and that is an act of care.

But because we are storytelling creatures, any ideas that we humans can have about stories are built upon and within the storytelling in which we *spin* our lives (McCarthy, 2007: 49–50). It is colloquial to talk about spinning a yarn, and that phrase deserves to be taken seriously. Humans spin the whole fabric of their lives through stories. When our stories are broken and inarticulate, the fabric of our lives is kinked, knotted, or torn. Where stories break off, incompletely told, a hole is torn in a life. Insofar as care aspires to make life whole, enhancing people's capacity to tell stories is a foundational act of caring. These ideas are expressed in scholarly and clinical literatures (Polkinghorne, 2004; M. White, 2007), but I *believe* these claims because they fit my understanding of my own story (Frank, 1991), which is to say, these claims are readily adaptable as a meta-narrative of my own storytelling.

If I were to make the arguments in this chapter without at least referencing my own storytelling, those arguments would be partially false. Until each of us – whether as clinician, or researcher, or human – begins with the clearest recognition of our own, personal need for storytelling, we remain ill equipped to offer the gift of our attention to the stories of others, and our analytical efforts to understand stories and storytelling, whatever value these efforts may have, will remain stunted.

This chapter focuses on two issues. First, what is the particular importance of storytelling for ill people? Stories, in my understanding, *work* for humans. Oxen cultivate fields, houses offer shelter; what kind of work can stories do for the ill? Behind the elaboration of the work that stories do is the clinical question of how those who care for the ill – whether professionals, volunteers, family, or friends – can best *attend* to stories. I choose this verb, *attend*, to suggest more than listening. To attend is to *be there*, in an existential as well as physical presence; that is, to be with another as if the lives of the person attending and the person being attended both depend on the quality of attention.

This chapter's second issue is what is *dangerous* about storytelling, a darker side that I did not give much attention to in my previous writing (Frank, 1995). Precisely because storytelling is powerful, it can damage. An analogy to pharmaceuticals is not misplaced: the right amount, at the right time, cures; the wrong amount, at the wrong time, sickens and even kills. Stories and storytelling are popular these days; narrative is in vogue. That popularity can lead to forgetting that if stories can be *helpers* – those characters, often small animals, who appear when the hero is desperate and offer what is necessary to continue the quest – stories are also *tricksters*, those characters around whom someone – often the trickster himself – gets hurt. Stories are not inherently benign. Their power is the complementary side of their danger.

How stories heal

In *The Wounded Storyteller* (Frank, 1995), I argued that illness is a *call for stories*. What is it specifically about storytelling as one way that people relate and connect, and about narrative as a form or structure that orders what is told, that can work for, with, and on the ill? The six benefits of storytelling that I propose are neither exhaustive nor are they mutually exclusive, but they begin to map a vast terrain.

First, the nature of narrative is to endow mere happenings with *shape and direction*, so that these happenings can become experience. I understand narrative (although I make no pretense of a definition) as *a representation of events in which one thing happens in consequence of another*. If one thing happens simply after another, with no apparent relation to what happened before, that is not yet narrative (H. White, 1973); or, in literary terms, there is no plot (Forster, 1954). We humans do not have experiences as spontaneous, natural occurrences. What we are able to know as experience, or, how we reduce and shape all that is happening into the narrower sphere known as experience, depends crucially on the stories that we already know. These stories teach us what sense to make of things – including relationships, other people, and material objects. They teach us to recognize which things are valuable (a loved one, a magic charm) and which are dangerous (a jealous sibling, a deceitful friend or even parent). Stories teach us how to respond to these things: a *plot* is a demonstration of which responses turn out well and which cause trouble. Experience may narrativize the world, but equally, narrative renders the world as able to be experienced.

Serious illness is one of those times in a life when things happen too fast to be assimilated into experience; events lack coherence, for several reasons. Sickness often disrupts the body's capacity to map its sensory experiences and to translate this mapping into what neurophysiologist Antonio Damasio (2000; 2003; see also Eakin, 2004) usefully calls the *movie-in-the-brain*, which is the beginning of human storytelling. The movie-in-the-brain *is* what we take to be the world we perceive: the world of continuous, flowing movements, in which each instant of perception is understood as following sequentially from the moment before and leading to the moment after. Pain, medications, and other effects of illness can disrupt the body's capacity to map itself and to produce a coherent movie-in-the-brain. Those of us who are old enough to recall moments in movie theatres when the projector jammed have a ready analogy. The smooth movement of the actors suddenly became jumpy; then the action stopped as the frame froze, and at worst, the screen went dark. Disease causes analogous effects. Storytelling works to restore the flow. Narrative repairs those moments of disruption of the movie-in-the-brain by restoring flow to a life's story, and with that flow, the coherence of things happening in consequence of recognized antecedent events and having predictable consequences.

If disease can physically disrupt people's narrative capacities, and thus their experiential capacities, a parallel disruption is caused by the institutions that offer treatment, but too often make this offer with a notable absence of generosity (Frank, 2004a). Entering these institutions requires that people becoming patients learn a new language: the medical vocabulary that describes symptoms, physiology, medications, and other treatment interventions. More difficult to learn is the institutional logic of what counts as care. Hospitals do not conceptualize care the way that uninstitutionalized people imagine being cared for. Hospitals understand it as perfectly normal to broadcast loud messages through corridors; hospitals consider it good care to wake patients up for all manner of purposes, however difficult sleep has been to achieve and however much it is needed; hospitals budget the time allocated to human contact; hospitals deprive the senses of natural light and of aesthetic pleasure . . . and this list could readily be extended far too long. Hospice and palliative care facilities work hard to minimize these institutional disruptions, but they remain institutions, with their own bureaucratic requirements and procedures (James and Field, 1992).

Being a patient also requires reorganizing normal human time and space. Hospital schedules – of procedures, examinations, and meals – are rarely geared to human needs. Hospital spaces require learning a new and complex geography of institutional spaces – spaces that compound the disorientations that physical ailment brings about. The disorientation of time and space requires a reorientation that narrative is distinctly prepared to offer, because stories, first and foremost, work to organize time and space (Bakhtin, 1981; Ricoeur, 1984). To *emplot* actions is to situate them in a temporality that narrative creates. As plots unfold in spaces, the unity of the plot gives those spaces coherence.

Telling good stories, in the sense of well-formed narratives, *restores coherence*, because narrative is a potent device for giving form to what becomes experience. That is what stories *do*: they shape what is inherently incoherent into what has a beginning, a middle, and an end, and one thing happens in consequence of something else. Especially when events in the story are terrible, narrative *serves* humans – again, it *works* for humans – by making what is terrible at least minimally graspable as having a comprehensible order.

Literary scholar Frank Kermode (1967) wrote that narrative *humanizes* time, in the sense of ordering time to make it habitable for humans. Narratives also humanize all the human terrors catalogued in Greek tragedy: a military leader sacrifices his daughter to bring favourable winds for the fleet; a hero goes mad and slaughters his children; another hero mistakenly kills his father and marries his mother. In rituals of dramatic tragedy, humans find a way to hold such events within a life that is truly terrifying, but that terror is humanized, in the sense of being rendered compatible with continuing human life. In the simplest terms, stories are the oldest, more enduring strategy by which we humans live with all that is incompatible with life. Stories are how we get on with it, over and against all that might stop us from persevering.

A second kind of work that stories do is to offer *distance* from the immediacy of events, and with this distance comes a degree of *choice* about the self one wants to be. By the *immediacy* of events I mean all that happens without buffering insulation; in a physiological metaphor, all that touches nerves that have been stripped of sheltering skin. How does narrative offer distance, or buffering? One of the insights of post-structuralist studies of narrative is to recognize the split between the 'I' of the narrator and the 'I' who is the subject of the narration (Belsey, 2002). Critic and storyteller Alberto Manguel (2007: 67) puts the issue clearly: 'Every story is a triangle made up of these binds: author and reader [or listener], reader and protagonist, protagonist and author'.

My own experience can clarify the healing potential of this separation between storyteller (Manguel's author) and protagonist. My memoir of my illnesses was published in 1991, and I began responding to requests to do public readings, an experience that had an unexpected effect on me. The story was still mine, but mine at a new distance. To tell a story in any form is to have to create a protagonist *as a character* who fits the narrative conventions of the story. In a first-person story, this protagonist is the storyteller him or herself, but as the story is told, a curious distancing begins to occur. The protagonist is me, truly enough, but me as I am *in that story*, or the *version* of me whom the story requires as its character. As a storyteller recognizes that the me-as-protagonist is created by choices from among a larger set of possible me's, then a sense of distance develops between the me to whom these things are happening and the me who is telling the tale. That protagonist is the poor fellow to whom these things happened, and may still be happening, while I, the storyteller, have the luxury of watching those things happen *to him*, at least so long as I go on telling his story.

This distancing effect does not imply dissociation. Instead, the lesson is that the complex work of associating a coherent self is always a work-in-progress or process. The self never just *is*, especially not during illness or trauma. Therein lies a crucial healing potential of storytelling. When I performed public readings from my memoir, *that* version became my experience. The subtitle of a recent collection of illness stories, *Women Write Their Bodies* (DasGupta and Hurst, 2007) expresses the same idea. Bodies, no less than experiences, are not naturally there, at least for consciousness. Bodies and experiences have to be *told into existence*.

The healing potential of telling life as a story lies in the twin palliatives of *distance* from the terrible immediacy of suffering, and *choice* about how to be a suffering self. Immediate suffering engulfs; it has no outside and offers no choices. Distance makes suffering less than total. Distance offers space outside suffering, or maybe through suffering. With more storytelling, life on the margins of suffering can develop, until that life can possibly balance the suffering, thus making it liveable.

The third kind of work that stories are singularly good equipments for doing is *expressing emotions* like anger that will fester if left unexpressed. One of the epigrams I chose for my own memoir expresses this contemporary belief in the necessity to express trauma. I quoted Christopher Durang, a popular playwright, who wrote in the director's notes to one of his plays: 'Unless you go through all the genuine angers you feel, both justified and unjustified, the feelings of love that you do have will not have any legitimate base and will be at least partially false. Plus, eventually you will go crazy' (Frank, 1991, front matter). Durang's claim has limits; in some times and places, people have not felt this need to 'go through' emotions such as anger. But I continue to believe that for many people, Durang expresses a psychological truth. Angers and resentments isolate people. This isolation compounds how *deep illness* (Frank, 1998) makes people feel alone. Stories work to bring people out of isolation; stories are *connectors* (Frank, 2004c), both medium and message of connection. To 'go through' angers by telling them in stories is to transform those angers into terms of connection.

The most frequent response of ill people to my memoir is that reading my story helped them to *feel less crazy*. I imagine other authors of illness narratives receiving the same message. Illness makes people feel crazy, in part, because others' responses make ill people question the legitimacy of their angers. An important, even crucial, prerequisite to feeling less crazy is for people to recognize that their angers are not theirs alone. Others had the same experiences and felt angry. But until stories connect these people, they question whether their angers are legitimate, and that questioning makes them feel crazy.

For those who offer care, stories that express anger may be the hardest to attend to. Caregivers often recognize themselves as implicated in the same acts about which the storyteller is expressing anger. For such listeners, the urge to question the legitimacy of those expressions of anger may be overwhelming. Moral courage can be required to recall the advice offered by Rachel Naomi Remen (1996: xxvii), who reminds caregivers that the emotional truth of a story, for the storyteller, is never the whole story of what happened. 'All real stories are true', Remen writes, even though there may be multiple stories that seem to contradict each other. 'All stories are full of bias and uniqueness, they mix fact with meaning' (xxxviii). What matters is to hear a person's story as the truth they need to tell in order to feel less alone and less crazy. And caregivers hearing angry stories can also remember that their stories also are what *they* need to feel less alone and less crazy, in their lives. Stories can remind everyone of the multiplicity of perspectives and realities that make life what it is.

Fourth, stories work to help people to regain a sense of *personal agency and responsibility* in their lives. Being a patient involves being acted upon. That may be a reality of one's physical condition, but it is no less limiting to one's character. Stories are driven forward on the strength of *character*, in the dual sense of characters as the players who act within the story, and *character* as the moral integrity of those individual characters. Plots generally hinge on some test of the character's character. Narrative worlds are places where character counts, because characters are *responsible* for what sort of thing happens after what else.

The act of telling one's story asserts the ill person's continuing capacity to assume responsibility for his or her life. The ultimate form of self-responsibility, when physical capacities may have been lost, can be interpretive responsibility.

Narrative form reasserts responsibility and moral sanity because within a plot, a character's actions have consequences. To borrow again Kermode's (1967) useful phrase, stories *humanize* amoral worlds by restoring the morality that can make such worlds fit places for human habitation – places in which action is human precisely because it involves individual responsibility.

Fifth, as many writers have asserted in many different forums, stories give humans the means to perform one of our crucial moral duties, which is *to witness* the suffering of others. Even when we humans can do nothing to relieve suffering, we can offer at least our presence (Frank, 1995; 1998; Kleinman, 1988; Remen, 1996). The offering of that presence is no small thing, no matter how immense the suffering is, and how much else is needed. I will not elaborate this point, but it may be the most important value of stories: a story connects the one who suffers with the one who has not known that suffering directly, in his or her body, but who can know it as mediated by the story, because of the shared vulnerability of our bodies. The connection continues when the witness tells the story.

Sixth and finally, stories help us humans to live with – never to unravel but at least live with – the mystery of our bodies. The paradoxical reality of bodies is that they provide humans' capacity for thought; as described earlier, the mapping of the body starts Damasio's (2000; 2003) movie-in-the-brain running; that movie-in-the-brain is *never anything more* than the body's mapping of itself. *But,* human bodies also exceed our capacity for thought. Bodies assert themselves, whether in pain, extreme performance, or joy, as an *excess* of what language or other symbols can express about it. During illness, bodies make themselves felt; sick bodies assert themselves (Leder, 1990), and bodies suddenly require speech (Frank, 1995). Illness is when the human limitation for articulating bodies can be frustrating. Stories, in common with aesthetic works, have the remarkable property of allowing people to say *more* than the literal words. Stories, like bodies, involve an excess, but this time the excess of signification over expression. Stories are literally excessive.

Ill people need stories to express as much as they can about these inexpressible, mysterious bodies, which have been the often unnoticed source of life, and then become the all too inescapable locus of dying. Death, as so many poets, philosophers, and scientists have written, marks the outer limit of the expressible. Stories with their tropes – their metaphors and other ways of pressing language beyond literal description – help people to *say more* than they thought themselves capable of articulating. Part of the aesthetic pleasure of stories comes from feeling allowed access to the limits of what can be said. But then, at some point in the best-told stories, narrative also allows the unsayable just to be, in its silence.

Those, then, are some values of stories and the work they can do, as human companions.

The dangers of narrative thinking

Stories work not only *for* humans, they also work *on* humans. I turn from how stories are helpers to how they are tricksters (Hyde, 1998; Radin, 1972). In using *trickster* as a trope, I emphasize here the destructive side of tricksters. Tricksters also give and create; like stories, tricksters have multiple, shifting sides. Stories can trick us humans into understanding our lives in ways that impede and damage those lives. Four dangers of stories seem especially significant: dangers of narrative form, genre problems, the susceptibility of stories to being means of coercion, and the moral insularity of stories. These dangers are not reasons to avoid stories, any more than the dangers of choking or poisoning are reasons to quit eating or drinking. The issue is how to be aware of the dangers and learn to live with them (Smith, 2005).

Narrative gives shape and direction to mere happenings by ordering these happenings within expected, recognizable forms or structures within which stories are told (Propp, 1968). Stories not only offer form to experience, they *impose* requirements of form on experience. One example of narrative form is that the quest of a protagonist requires the opposition of an antagonist; lacking that opposition, the story will not generate suspense, and without suspense, a recounting of events is scarcely a story. Recreating a life as a story can require conscripting someone or something to be the antagonist. The antagonistic tendencies of some person or some personified process may have to be exaggerated – narrative form demands no less. In mainstream medicine narratives, death is often conscripted as the ultimate antagonist (Rieff, 2008). Palliative care, which in principle accepts death as a natural part of life, expends considerable effort to undo this conventional idea, both medical and lay, of death as the ultimate antagonist that must be tricked or defeated. As long as death is the antagonist, then dying will be a kind of defeat, which is an unhappy way to die.

Narrative thinking also requires obstacles as tests of character. Because many stories take the form of quests – a hero seeking some desired object, which may be a person (the loved one), a thing (the Holy Grail), or completion of a task (slaying the dragon) – narrative thinking embeds the idea that obstacles must be overcome for there to be a closure. Moreover, obstacles are necessarily understood as a personal *test*, conveying a sense of individual victory or defeat. The risk here is that narrative thinking can create obstacles where there are none. Stories easily trick us humans into feeling tested by what may be nothing more than how things are; the nature of bodies is to wear out; eventually, people die. A worn out body can be an obstacle, but it is not necessarily a test. Death is only participation in a cycle that bodies were designed for. Stories become tricksters when they lead people to invent antagonistic forces and to expend limited energy seeking to overcome these forces. A helper story reasserts the ease of accepting a nature beyond narrative: autumn is not a test for the leaves; only a personified leaf struggles to cling to the branch.

A second trickster danger of stories is the narrative requirement of making *genre* choices. Emotional and cognitive reactions to what happens in stories depend on how listeners understand the genre of the story; that is, the recognizable type of story, with attendant expectations not only for how those actions are understood and responded to. In a comedy, slipping on a banana peel is funny, because in that genre, injuries do not incur actual suffering; characters fall but are not hurt; exaggerated expressions of pain bring more laughter. In the tragedy of *Oedipus Rex*, the irony of Oedipus seeking the man who killed the former King – when the audience knows he himself is that man – is not funny, although irony can be comic when the genre is comedy. Illness can be an occasion for *genre conflicts*, when different people seek to assert their way of understanding what kind of story they all are living.

Mutual frustration is assured when participants in any storytelling make different genre choices. The more serious the illness, the more participants' interpretations are mutually dependent, and the more genre differences will grate, becoming conflicts. For example, and stereotypically, a physician may understand the story as a sequence of riddle-like puzzles, in which each discrete symptom requires a treatment solution, and death comes as a surprise (Cassell, 2000). Others attending a dying person – and much of my work has encouraged this genre choice – can understand the story as a romance, in which the hero's character develops through overcoming a sequence of obstacles, which may be internal or external. The mastery achieved by a dying hero is often expressed symbolically by the person's capacity to choose the timing of death (Callanan and Kelley, 1993; Remen, 1996). By contrast, a comic genre choice is expressed by some very ill patients who use phrases like 'having a good sense of humour' or 'keeping it light' to describe qualities they value. They express a commitment to treating their impending death as a comedy. None of these genre choices can be wrong, in itself. The dangers can be failing to recognize either the effect that genre choices have on others, especially long-term bereavement effects, or failing to recognize the commitment that others have to a different genre choice.

People's genre choices represent deep commitments, and these choices appear so self-evidently necessary to those who hold them that they are difficult to discuss, much less to change (Taylor, 1989). Too often, genre choices turn into a contest over who can sustain his or her choice for how long, against what level of explicit opposition by others who want to tell a different kind of story. The timing and appropriateness of referral to palliative care can be a contest over genre choices, and the tenacity with which people hold to their chosen type of story is evident. Hospice and palliative care institutions are no exceptions to the general tendency of all institutions to assert what genre choices they prefer their clients or patients to uphold (Frank, 2004b). Working against this pervasive tendency of any institution requires constant self-reflection and interrogation of received therapeutic beliefs.

A third danger of stories, and an especially prevalent danger in contemporary health care, is that storytelling can be hijacked – appropriated and regulated – by institutional interests that want particular stories told in circumscribed ways, in order to advance a specific agenda. As much as I have emphasized the validity of the quest narrative as a response to serious illness (Frank, 1995), I am made nervous by the rhetorical regularity of these stories in newsletters published in North American support-groups. The conventional rhetoric of these stories requires that any losses from illness be transformed into unambiguous 'gifts'. Authors join in lockstep expressions of unqualified gratitude for 'all that cancer has brought into my life'. At the extreme, some health charities script ill people's stories for more effective use as marketing devices for fund-raising (King, 2006). Loss and ongoing sadness, recognition of how disease can diminish life, have no place in this triumphal narrative form (Conway, 2007). This phenomenon is not unique to health care. Studies of diverse recovery groups (Holstein and Gubrium, 2000; Irvine, 1999) demonstrate how membership involves learning to tell one's story within an evaluative template that is acceptable to the group, including emotional modulation.

A final danger of stories is their tendency towards moral insularity. Sometimes, reality is tautological: stories make sense within groups of people whose conception of *what* makes sense has been shaped by the particular stories that are understood in shared ways within those groups. That narrative sharing is a crucial factor in what makes a collection of people worth calling a group. This issue is expressed by anthropologist Julie Cruikshank (1990), in her ethnographic study of Yukon women elders who were master storytellers. Cruikshank quotes Angela Sidney, one of these elders, saying: 'I want to live my life right, just like a story.' Angela Sidney's face, as it appears on the cover of the book, seems an iconic image of wisdom: it suggests all the experience and kindness that would be associated with being an *elder*.

Yet, there is a substantial problem with what Angela Sidney says: she elides the questions of *which* stories teach people how to live their lives right, and who gets to assert the proper understanding of these stories, especially their implications for action. For example, people who join movements to achieve justice and equality seek to live their lives right, and they tell some story as showing them what counts as right (Davis, 2002; Polletta, 2006), but social movements take sides on contested issues. Those outside the movement deny that the movement's stories actually represent events as they happened. Other groups' stories place the events in different plots that begin with different precipitating events and show characters as having different motivations. These people also claim to be living their lives right, according to different stories, differently understood.

At the end of life, everyone wants a good death, just like a story they have heard – and that is the problem. People have been compelled by different stories, telling different versions of what a good death is. Those who affiliate around some particular story can become insular in asserting this story as the privileged template for the treatment and care of the dying person.

In palliative care, both the family of the dying person and the care-giving team are at risk of moral insularity, as they sustain particular features of a 'good death' narrative and then attribute paramount importance to enacting those features. These features can include, but are by no means limited to: reconciliations of old animosities, spiritual realization, physical presence of certain loved ones (and maybe others' absence), display of certain emotions (and not others), striking a particular balance between pain and lucidity, and expression of preferred attitudes about death, including what regrets or complaints can be voiced by whom. People can be so deeply grounded in how these features are supposed to be present in a 'good death' that self-reflection can be difficult to achieve.

Chaos breaks out when events undercut the possibility of the preferred story being realized, or when some participants have established commitments to different stories. Some families may have cohesive 'good death' narratives, developed through a history of family deaths as these are remembered in stories of what went well or badly. But in other families, geographical and other divergences may have led members to different narrative preferences. Religions were once primary sources of good-death narratives, but today, popular culture may be the most potent narrative resource for many people. Palliative care teams evolve their own 'good death' narrative, based on shared clinical experience, professional training, both explicit and tacit recognitions of certain institutional necessities, personal commitments that initially drew workers to palliative care, as well as their own family narratives. A good death may be one in which everyone imagines enacting the same story; the crucial clinical task is to approximate that alignment as closely as possible.

The Yukon elder Angela Sidney is certainly right: humans do learn through stories much if not all of what they believe about living a life right. But she does not say that people learn from different stories, and even within different groups the same stories can be understood differently, especially the moral implication of the story. She does not say that people have often learned their stories too well, so that other stories sound wrong at best and less than human at worst. She does not say that if stories are humans' indispensable helpers, they are also tricksters getting us into such characteristic troubles as creating adversity where there may be none, misunderstanding what kind of story we find ourselves in, taking up those stories in which others want our lives to be told, and becoming insular as we uphold what we take to be the moral truth of our stories.

Stories and palliative care

Where, then, does this leave practices of palliative care, with respect to stories and storytelling? Most simply put, dying needs stories because dying confronts humans with what is most strange and unpredictable; dying, perhaps more than anything else that humans confront, requires being humanized. Stories bridge principles of how to act with practicalities of taking action. Patients and families find themselves having to translate principles they believe in (or thought they believed in) with practical decisions they now face. For health care workers, institutional or professional standards of practice – guidelines for good care – have to be translated into the practicalities of clinical action, in situations where so much can be happening simultaneously that more than one guideline or principle seems to apply.

The clinical problem is that even the most generally agreed-upon objective – for example, that people should not be in pain – is not so unambiguous in practice. Preventing pain often involves compromising a person's other abilities, ultimately consciousness itself (Byock, 1997: 193–216). Stories situate principles, rules, and guidelines in practical action. As one thing happens in consequence of something else, stories show how different actions turn out for better or worse. Stories *teach* on an affective and even corporeal level that principles, rules, and guidelines cannot. But then the dangerous side of story reappears: people become committed to one story as the privileged understanding and guide to what is happening.

The best and perhaps the only remedy to the dangers of stories is *openness* to more stories. If narrative form requires and thus creates antagonists and obstacles, it is possible to tell other stories in which characters come to realize that the obstacles they believed in are more the products of their own imaginations than actual realities. When genre choices limit people's understanding of what kind of a story can be told, the best way to open their choices is with a different story in a different genre. When people seem to be captured by an imposed way of telling their story – not simply caught up, as all of us are in good stories – but *captured* as a shutting down of alternatives, they can still hear a story about someone who explores alternatives, perhaps of emotional expression, that are beyond the rhetorical limits of the imposed story. And finally, the most effective way to begin to open the moral insularity of people's commitment to *their* stories is to offer them not criticisms of those stories and the stance they encourage, but simply to offer other stories of other people. But why should people take up this offer of stories? Why should these counter-narratives (Nelson, 2001) be effective?

I have left out what may be the most important feature of stories: they depend on and they inspire *imagination*, and humans are imaginative creatures. A story, unlike a code, guideline, or principle, asks first that the listener imagine. That imaginative opening is the story's appeal, and it is why people who may be closed to other forms of argument just might be willing to listen to a story. Or, they might be willing to tell their own story again, adding a new detail this time, and if their attention is called to that detail and to different ways of understanding it, their story might change.

The clinical commitment is to support, so far as possible, at least three aspects of people's storytelling. First, people need support in choosing *well* what stories they tell about their lives and in their lives, in a world that not only presents but often aggressively markets so many stories for taking up as one's own. Second, in a world where others seek to limit people's interpretive possibilities, people need to be reminded that they are making interpretive decisions about how they understand these stories; they are deciding what counts, in a story, as choosing and acting *well*. Third, people have a duty to reflect on the consequences of their stories not only for their own lives, but also as these stories affect the lives of those around them.

The delicate balance of clinical work is how gently or how hard to push people off one story and towards another. The narrative clinician's skill is to offer stories that open new possible stories, without seeming to push at all.

References

Bakhtin, M. M. (1981) *The Dialogic Imagination: Four Essays.* University of Texas Press, Austin, TX.

Belsey, C. (2002) *Poststructuralism: A Very Short Introduction.* Oxford, New York.

Byock, I. (1997) *Dying Well: The Prospect for Growth at the End of Life.* Riverhead Books, New York.

Callanan, M. and Kelley, P. (1993) *Final Gifts: Understanding the Special Awareness, Needs, and Communications of the Dying.* Bantam Books, New York.

Cassell, E. J. (2000) The principles of the Belmont report revisited: How have respect for persons, beneficence, and justice been applied in clinical medicine? *Hastings Center Report*, **30**(4), 12–21.

Conway, K. (2007) *Illness and the Limits of Expression*. University of Michigan Press, Ann Arbor, MI.

Cruikshank, J. (1990) *Life Lived Like a Story*. University of British Columbia Press, Vancouver.

Cruikshank, J. (1998) *The Social Life of Stories: Narrative and Knowledge in the Yukon Territory*. University of Nebraska Press, Lincoln, NE.

Damasio, A. (2000) *The Feeling of What Happens: Body, Emotion, and the Making of Consciousness*. Vintage, New York.

Damasio, A. (2003) *Looking for Spinoza: Joy, Sorrow, and the Feeling Brain*. Harcourt, Inc., New York.

DasGupta, S. and Hurst, M. (eds) (2007) *Stories of Illness and Healing: Women Write Their Bodies*. The Kent State University Press, Ken, OH.

Davis, J.E. (ed.) (2002) *Stories of Change: Narrative and Social Movements*. State University of New York Press, Albany, NY.

Eakin, P. J. (2004). What are we reading when we read autobiography? *Narrative*, **12**, 121–32.

Forster, E. M. (1954) *Aspects of the Novel*. Harcourt, Brace, and World, New York.

Frank, A. W. (1991) *At the Will of the Body: Reflections on Illness*. Houghton Mifflin, Boston.

Frank, A. W. (1995) *The Wounded Storyteller: Body, Illness, and Ethics*. The University of Chicago Press, Chicago.

Frank, A. W. (1998) Just listening: narrative and deep illness. *Families, Systems and Health*, **16**, 197–212.

Frank, A. W. (2004a) *The Renewal of Generosity: Illness, Medicine, and How to Live* The University of Chicago Press, Chicago.

Frank, A. W. (2004b) Narratives of spirituality and religion in end-of-life care. In *Narrative Research in Health and Illness* (eds. B.Hurwitz, T. Greenhalgh and V. Skultans). Blackwell Publishing, Malden, MA and Oxford. pp. 132–45.

Frank, A. W. (2004c) Health stories as connectors and subjectifiers. *Health: An Interdisciplinary Journal for the Social Study of Health, Illness, and Medicine*, **10**, 421–40.

Holstein, J.A. and Gubrium, J. F. (2000) *The Self We Live By: Narrative Identity in a Postmodern World*. Oxford, New York.

Hyde, L. (1998) *Trickster Makes This World*. North Point Press, New York.

Irvine, L. (1999) *Codependent Forevermore: The Invention of Self in a Twelve Step Group*. University of Chicago Press, Chicago.

James, N. and Field, D. (1992) The routinization of hospice: charisma and bureaucratization. *Social Science and Medicine*, **34**(12), 1363–75.

Kermode, F. (1967) *The Sense of an Ending: Studies in the Theory of Fiction*. Oxford, New York.

King, S. (2006) *Pink Ribbons, Inc.: The Politics of Breast Cancer*. University of Michigan Press, Ann Arbor MI.

Kleinman, A. (1988) *The Illness Narratives: Suffering, Healing, and the Human Condition*. Basic Books, New York.

Leder, D. (1990) *The Absent Body*. University of Chicago Press, Chicago.

McCarthy, J. (2007) *Dennett and Ricoeur on the Narrative Self*. Humanity Books, Amherst, NY.

MacIntyre, A. (1984) *After Virtue*. Notre Dame University Press, Notre Dame, IN.

Manguel, A. (2007) *The City of Words*. ON, Anansi, Toronto.

Nelson, H. L. (2001) *Damaged Identities, Narrative Repair*. Cornell University Press, Ithaca, NY.

Polkinghorne, D. E. (2004) *Practice and the Human Sciences: The Case for a Judgment-Based Practice of Care*. State University of New York Press, Albany, NY.

Polletta, F. (2006) *It Was Like a Fever: Storytelling in Protest and Politics*. University of Chicago Press, Chicago.

Propp, V. (1968) *Morphology of the Folktale*. University of Texas Press, Austin, TX.

Radin, P. (1972) *The Trickster: A Study in American Indian Mythology*. Schocken Books, New York.

Remen, R. (1996) *Kitchen Table Wisdom: Stories That Heal*. Riverhead Books, New York.

Ricoeur, P. (1984) *Time and Narrative, Volume 1*. University of Chicago Press, Chicago.

Rieff, D. (2008) *Swimming in a Sea of Death: A Son's Memoir*. Simon and Schuster, New York.

Smith, P. (2005) *Why War? The Cultural Logic of Iraq, The Gulf War, and Suez*. The University of Chicago Press, Chicago.

Taylor, C. (1989) *The Sources of the Self: The Making of the Modern Identity*. Harvard University Press, Cambridge, MA.

White, H. (1973) *Metahistory: The Historical Imagination in Nineteenth Century Europe*. Johns Hopkins University Press, Baltimore, MD.

White, M. (2007) *Maps of Narrative Practice*. Norton, New York.

Chapter 11

Life story and life review

Irene Renzenbrink

> I was born, I grew up, I studied, I loved, I married,
> I procreated, I said, I wrote, all gone now. I went, I saw,
> I did… I'm getting somewhere now, I'm feeling lighter.
> I'm coming unstuck from albums, from diaries, from
> journals, from space and time. Only a paragraph left,
> only a sentence or two, only a whisper.
> I was born.
> I was.
> I.
>
> Margaret Attwood, *Life Stories* (2006: 5)

For some people it may well be just as Margaret Attwood suggests in one of her more stringent short stories about reminiscence. No fuss, no drama, just a few facts and figures. For others, particularly in this age of self-disclosure, there will be a need to share their life in greater detail, in all its drama and complexity. Some people are pragmatic, rational, and well defended. Others are more expressive and willing to expose their vulnerability. In working with people at the end of their lives, the important thing to remember is that it is their story, not ours, and they have a right to tell as much or as little in whichever manner they choose. Some people die never having shared their warts-and-all life story. How often do we say that we have learned more about a person at their funeral than we ever knew during their lifetime?

Having said that, we also know that hospice and palliative care often provides a setting in which caring and skilled staff establish special bonds with patients. Through a process which Kleinman (1988) refers to as 'empathic witnessing', patients may feel safe, heard, and understood and life stories may be shared willingly and with positive outcomes. For example, Lester (2005) refers to the empowering effects of life review for clients who are terminally ill and how the knowledge gained during the process can help with assessment and care plans. She has documented the benefits of life review with hospice patients in alleviating emotional distress, reaffirming identity and self-worth and bringing renewed physical emotional energy despite limited life expectancy.

In the following discussion, I provide a broad overview of life story and life review work, highlighting practical methods and models that have been used in different disciplinary settings and internationally. I draw particular attention to the emotional challenges of such work, the need for staff to receive special training, supervision, and support and the need to remain cautious about the increasing technology surrounding reminiscence at the end of life. My engagement with this broader literature is grounded in my experiences of applying a life review exercise to my own experiences of illness and caring.

Concepts and approaches

Life story work is a term given to biographical approaches in health and social care that give people the opportunity to narrate their life experiences. It involves using this life story to benefit them in their present situation (McKeown et al. 2006). There is a growing body of knowledge about life story and life review work with different social groups such as those living with AIDS, intellectually disabled people, people suffering from dementia and Alzheimer's disease, and older people living in nursing homes, as well as with hospice and palliative care patients.

However, a systematic literature review on the subject (McKeown et al. 2006: 238) found that there is 'no commonly accepted definition, approach or outcome in life story work'. A number of gaps in research were identified including the lack of comparison of various life review methods and their merits, insufficient engagement with the user's experience and the impact on staff attitudes where people sharing their stories lived in institutional settings.

According to Kunz (2002) the difficulties in formulating an overall conceptual framework may be related to the fact that the field is multidisciplinary with many different methods and applications in use. A list of life story work activities might include recording and writing life stories, scrapbooking, reminiscence groups, formal oral history and even quilting, blogging, and online diaries (Kunz, 2002). In the field of child protection there has even been a marriage of life story work with scrapbooking tenets and techniques called 'scrapathy' (Bayliss, 2007). No wonder there is some confusion and concern about quality!

Origins of the life review concept

As Kunz (2002) explains, the term 'life review' was first coined by pioneering gerontologist Robert Butler in 1955 when he identified life review as a normal aspect of adult development. Having spent time with what he described as 'vibrant older people' and later patients in both individual and group therapy, Butler (2002: 1) concluded that 'life review is a normal function of the later years and not a pathological condition'. He defined life review as 'a personal process by which a person evaluates his or her life as it nears its end. Memories, reminiscence and nostalgia all play a part in the process'. Rather than being considered as the irrelevant babble of older people, life review came to be seen as having a significant and positive role with therapeutic value. Butler (2002: 2) believed that life review was a natural healing process which could result in 'the righting of old wrongs, making up with estranged family members or friends, coming to accept one's mortality, gaining a sense of serenity, pride in accomplishment, and a feeling of having done one's best'.

The main purpose of life review for an older person is to achieve what Erikson described as a 'sense of coherence and wholeness', thus resolving the final developmental crisis in adulthood: the crisis of 'integrity vs despair'. (Kunz and Soltys, 2007). According to Erikson's theorizing, successful resolution of this crisis results in an attitude of 'acceptance of self, both past and present' and the emergence of personal wisdom. However, there is also the possibility of the opposite outcome and of being left in 'despair' with unresolved feelings of guilt, doubt, and remorse. Haight (2001) describes life review as a soul-searching or meaning-making process through which individuals learn to evaluate, integrate, and accept life as it has been lived. It is through this process that they learn to approach death with greater equanimity. It is generally agreed that the process is best served when shared with a caring and non-judgmental listener. Haight (2001: 1) also emphasizes the value of sharing life stories with caring understanding people because 'sharing one's inner thoughts, shameful moments and secret prides in such a manner is an act of intimacy, for both the listener and the teller'.

This is not unlike the *anam cara* relationship, to which philosopher and poet, John O'Donohue (1998) referred in his writings on Celtic wisdom and spirituality. He wrote: 'It originally referred to someone who acted as a teacher, companion and spiritual guide . . . someone to whom you confessed, revealing the hidden intimacies of your life. With the *anam cara* you could share your innermost self, your mind and your heart. The superficial and functional lies and half truths of social acquaintance fall away, you can be as you really are' (p. 13).

Life story work in social care

Life story work and life review in hospice and palliative care has much in common with other fields of social care such as intellectual disability and foster care because of common philosophical commitments and the importance of validating difficult life experiences.

The development of life story work with intellectually disabled people in The Netherlands is described by Meininger (2006: 181) as a 'reaction against practices which are purely functional and instrumental within a diagnosis-treatment model'. It is argued that life story work enables disabled people to better express themselves and to advocate more effectively on their own behalf. In reviewing the literature on life story work Meininger found three types of life story. First, there is the *chronicle*, a chronologically ordered listing of facts and data that charts the story of the person's life, usually written by a professional. This seems to be quite similar to a care plan as the information gathered helps to formulate person-centred goals of care.

Second, a *life book or memory book* containing information about events, persons, and objects that are of importance to the disabled person and typically including photos and mementoes. This kind of story book usually remains in the person's possession and is similar to those developed with children in the field of foster care and adoption to maintain a sense of order and continuity in an otherwise fragmented life.

A third approach consists of *life stories*, described as narrative compositions based on selected experiences of the person with learning disabilities or an autobiography that charts the person's whole life. The key feature is that the individuality of the person is expressed in a coherent fashion, capturing their unique identity and character. This view helps to break down prejudices and misunderstandings and is seen as empowering for the disabled person.

Life story work in the field of adoption and foster care is a method used to record the child or young person's history and personal development and assist them to develop a sense of self in relation to their life experiences. It is described as a 'valuable process in enabling children/young people to feel connected with significant people and places, their family of origin and their heritage' (Foster Care Associates).

The use of life story books is a well-established practice in working with children and young people in foster care and emphasizes the uniqueness of each child's life, the power of story and the importance of working hard to 'put together the bits and pieces of your life into one story – the good bits and the bad bits' (British Association of Adoption and Foster Care). A life story book is described as a 'collection of information and memorabilia collected by and for a child or young person whose life has involved multiple placements and/or trauma to enable the child or young person to make sense of their past' (The United Kingdom Social Care Association). With the help of a skilled facilitator or counsellor children are given an opportunity to write about their strengths, survival skills, and their capacity to grow and change.

The focus is on the production of a book or written record of the child's family history, likes and dislikes, school achievements, friends, pets and hobbies, and other matters of interest to them. The book remains in the possession of the child who is encouraged to keep it in a safe place. Letters to teachers, parents, and caregivers may be included. Sometimes a box decorated with colourful pictures and glitter is used as a container for the book and special objects, photos, and mementoes. These are similar to the Memory Boxes that are often used by bereaved children to maintain their connection to a deceased relative or friend. As Rossouw (2003: 2) explains, 'a life story book can help with identity formation, assist in resolving separation issues, help build trust in adults, resolve strong emotions linked to past events, help separate fact and fantasy, and identify both positive and negative aspects of family lives'.

Life review in palliative care

Technical explanations flatten the story of my illness.

(Broyard, 1992: 66)

While there are a number of theoretical perspectives and practices associated with life story work and life review in the human services field, there are particular issues and challenges in applying these concepts to the field of palliative care.

For many people living with a life-threatening or incurable illness, it is more than likely that the stories they tell are stories about their illness, or as Arthur Frank (2002) writes:

> What most ill persons say about their illness comes from their physicians and other medical staff, not from themselves. The ill person as patient is simply repeating what has been said elsewhere-boring second hand medical talk. When ill persons try to talk in medicalese, they deny themselves the drama of their personal experience. (p. 4)

The whole-person approach – the hallmark of palliative care – recognizes that there is much more to a patient's experience of illness than symptoms and treatment. However, even in hospice and palliative care services, where the focus and stated philosophy is about the person with the disease rather than the disease itself, the physical care and control of pain and distressing symptoms may well claim greater staff attention at times. The pressure of limited resources will also affect the range of services offered and staff may not always have the time, sensitivity, and special training required for the tasks of life story work and life review with dying patients. If this work is to be carried out with skill and commitment it must be first supported by management so that protocols for the protection of privacy and confidentiality can be developed. One of the obstacles that McKeown et al. (2006) identified in reviewing a number of life story work programmes was the lack of management support and investment in staff support and training.

In an introduction to 'Lifestory', a life story guide book produced by The Irish Hospice Foundation (2006), John Waters writes:

> Sometimes in our concentration on what our life is like now, we can miss the richness to be unearthed in the multiplicity of days behind us. The different phases we have been through as human beings. The places where we have lived or been. The people we have known or become close to. The things that have happened to us, the significance of which only reveals itself with time. And beyond that, the stories that led to our presence here in the first place; our antecedents and their hopes and dreams, their thoughts and deeds, their loves and losses. (p. 18)

In *Dying to Know, Bringing Death to Life*, produced by Pilotlight Australia (2007) we are introduced to an older woman called Mary, 'who has done a lot of things that no one ever asks her about'. Mary is typical of so many frail older people who become invisible in a materialistic and youth-oriented society. Some of her life story and essence is captured in the following extract:

> Mary was born just after World War I in country New South Wales. She was the school high jump champion and competed in the state finals. She used to ride to school on her horse with both her brothers on board. They laughed all the way there most mornings, until Terry fell off and broke his arm. Mary trained as a nurse and worked in London during the blitzkrieg. She met the prime minister Robert Menzies once. And Dawn Fraser. She preferred Dawn Fraser. She only marched in protest once because she didn't want her sons conscripted. Her favourite dance is the samba, which she is still pretty good at.

This example shows that life story work can be whimsical, light hearted and brief, while also conveying chronology and biographical meaning. Perhaps creativity and a touch of irreverence are also needed at times. Older people and people facing the end of life will contribute their own creative efforts with artistic work, prose, and poetry.

A well-known example can be found in the poem 'What do you see, nurse?' also known as The Crabbit Old Woman, attributed to Phyllis McCormack (Kunz and Soltys, 2007) and said to be found among the possessions of a nursing home resident in Scotland after her death. The poem reminds us to acknowledge the whole life story of a person who is frail, seriously ill, disabled, or dying. The old woman in the poem asks the nurse to look beyond her crumbling body and reviews her life as a small child, a young girl, a bride, a mother, a widow, and grandmother. She writes:

> But inside this old carcass a young girl still dwells,
> And now and again my battered heart swells.
> I remember the joys, I remember the pain,
> And I'm loving and living life over again.

While reminiscence, life review, and life story work will have benefits, the emotional impact for both the teller and the listener should not be underestimated. As Lester (2005: 76) reminds us, 'bringing oneself, as a professional, into a relationship at the end of a person's life can be a daunting prospect. When David Oliviere (2002) wrote about his relationship with Sarah, a 75-year-old patient who entrusted him with the care of her cat, Pickles, he said, 'Her situation resurrected for me the issues of pets, openness and cancer, and fondness. All my life was there before me' (p. 103).

Support, guidance, and supervision for staff working with patients in an intensive and structured way will ensure that stories are gathered with empathy and sensitivity and that the worker will maintain the necessary energy levels and enthusiasm for the task. If staff feel overwhelmed and anxious in the face of death they might begin to avoid emotionally charged areas of discussion. It is equally important to 'start where the client is' and work at a pace that is acceptable and comfortable for them. According to Australian researcher Beverley Raphael (1984) the capacity for compassion or 'suffering together with another' allows us to 'empathize with the distress of others and to offer them comfort and consolation'. She goes on to say:

> Empathy with the dying and the bereaved may bring distress for us, proportionate to the severity of their loss, the closeness of our identification with their situation, and the degree to which our own earlier pain has been revived. (p. 404)

Raphael also recommends the use of supervision and support from other workers, family, and friends. Without comfort, consolation, and time away from stressful encounters the worker may run the risk of burn out or may develop distancing and dehumanizing behaviours (see Menzies Lyth, 1988).

The use of life review frameworks

An English example

The structured life review approach used by English hospice social worker, Jennie Lester, in her work with people facing death, is based on Barbara Haight's *Life Review and Experiencing Form* developed and tested with older people in the 1980s (Lester, 2005). As Lester explains, the structured life review 'encourages the exploration of a person's life by means of sensitizing questions, covering the main themes of a person's life, provided in a one-to-one relationship built on confidentiality and trust (p. 69). The life review questionnaire is given to the patient or client one week before the first planned session and three sessions are then conducted to explore the themes of childhood/family life, adulthood/work life, and the 'here and now'.

These life story sessions go beyond the kind of social history taking and psycho-social assessment that is commonly used in palliative care and health care generally. Lester's compelling case-study examples show marked improvement in levels of emotional well-being, family relationships, and preparedness for the process of dying and death.

A New Zealand example

An extension of the life review approach has been developed at Te Omanga Hospice in Lower Hutt, New Zealand in a 'biography as therapy' programme. Trained volunteers assist patients and their families to compile written and oral biographies (Lichter, 1993). While there has not been a formal evaluation of the programme it is the perception of staff that the biography has been a key factor in improving a patient's mood and sense of well-being. Life review is seen as a tool for the discovery of meaning in a patient's life and this in turn helps them to face their dying and death with greater equanimity.

The 'biographers' are volunteer members of the family support team and are carefully selected, trained, supervised, and supported in their work. They have meetings with an experienced oral historian and with a journalist who special-izes in biographical outlines and advice is given on interviewing techniques (Lichter, 1993). After establishing rapport with the patient, the volunteer tapes the conversations and then produces a written record for presentation to the patient and or family. Sessions obviously have to be tailored to the patient's level of strength and well-being. It is the experience of the hospice staff that almost without exception the offer to do a biography has been accepted with enthusiasm and it is the feeling of patients, relatives, and staff that the collation of such biographies helps in the restoration of meaning and purpose to lives.

A Canadian example

Canadian palliative care physician and author of *What Dying People Want* (2002), David Kuhl provides a detailed and helpful guide for conducting a life review with dying people, based on a structure proposed by gerontologists Birren et al. (1995). The life review process begins with a reflection of the major 'branching points' or significant events in the patient's life. Kuhl (2002) defines life review as 'simply living in the present while looking at the past. It enables the individual to reconsider life events, relationships, successes, failures. It may also remind the person of conversations and activities that might still be desirable' (p. 31).

The branching points developed in Birren, Deutchman and DeVries's 'guided autobiography' include family of origin, career and life's work, the role of money, health and body image, aspirations, life goals and meaning of life, loves and hates, sexual identity and experiences, and grief. Kuhl states that life review is 'more than merely remembering or reminiscing' and that 'grief is often part of the process of looking back over one's life story' (p. 156). Life review may also spark a search for meaning as an individual tries to make sense of confusing and difficult experiences and remembers many significant events involving loss and change. In this way there is a significant area of overlap between life story work and the work of grief and mourning, which has been described by Parkes as a kind of emotional nostalgia in bereavement: 'As time passes, if all goes well, the intensity of pining diminishes and the pain and pleasure of recollection are experienced as a bittersweet mixture of emotions, "nostalgia"' (Personal Communication, 2008).

Kuhl (2002) speaks about 'bearing witness to the experience of living and dying with a terminal illness'. He emphasizes the need to 'be with' the person who is ill and of really hearing what is being said. Doctors and other health care professionals are trained to assess and judge what patients are saying and therefore need to 'stop being detectives' and learn to listen 'not only with their ears but with their heart as well'.

Whiting and Bradley (2007) refer to the 'artful witnessing' involved in the 'sacred and vulnerable process of constructing and reconstructing a life story in the hope of creating a sense of integrity about one's life as it has been lived' (p.127); their work with older adults they aim to synthesize the concepts of life review; Erikson's (1963) ego integrity and narrative reconstruction and drawing in particular on Neimeyer's (2001) model of meaning reconstruction in grief and bereavement. Their life review work therefore attempts to help people makes sense of and discover the benefits in their difficult experiences, and forge a new identity by incorporating the loss into their life story.

The following story was written by Dr Frank Brennan, a palliative care physician from Sydney, Australia who has also worked in a hospice in Ireland. It captures the beauty of a helping encounter in which he offers advice and information while at the same time, respecting the wishes of the patient's wife. His careful listening as she shares the story of their life together is a fine example of 'artful witnessing' (Whiting and Bradley, 2007) at a time of vulnerability:

The Woman from County Meath

The warmth of the Dublin day caught everyone by surprise. Through the window I could see children playing in the garden. We had walked into the visitors' room. The family was waiting. They were from County Meath. He was a farmer, only 54. She was a teacher. They had seven children. It was clear that he was dying. He had battled seemingly intractable pain, but now over the past few days was much more settled. I spoke about these days and what to expect from this point onwards. I then concentrated on the family themselves and recommended, as we do, the usual things –that they each take turns in being with him, that they try to eat and sleep, that they talk to each other, in short to look after themselves through this vigil. I turned to the patient's wife and said, 'I know you've been here all the time over the last few days. It might be good to go and have a rest, even just for a little while.' There was a long silence. She looked at me as though down a passage. She turned her head to one side, looked out the window, then towards me again and said, 'No, I will not be leaving him.' She spoke tenderly of their first meeting at age of 17, of their courting and their wedding day, of their marriage and the birth of their children. She spoke in soft beautiful phrases, then sentences that began plainly, but became brilliant, each seemingly more evocative than the last. And with every memory of their life together, each reflection she would end by saying, 'No, I will not be leaving him', until that phrase became the tolling of a distant bell.

And then she said something that I have never heard expressed in the same way before. She said that from their wedding day they were united, that they were as the prayer states, one body, and that as he had fallen ill, so had she, that as he was buffeted by the storms of pain, so was she, that as he was suffering, so was she, and that as he lay dying, so was she. No James Joyce, no Oscar Wilde, no Samuel Beckett could have put it so powerfully. As Angela Murphy, the palliative care nurse with me in the room that day said later, 'She was saying what he was feeling.'

In many ways she was not talking to us. She was speaking across the vast sea of their lives. I had spoken at a practical level about rest. The response I received was from a person adrift on that sea, not wanting to leave or soften the fate. Too often, as doctors, we speak practically and are heard emotionally. And, perhaps, that is our role. Angela and I left the room and walked back to the ward. We were both too moved to say much. Later that day Angela rang me and said, Frank, we may never hear the like of that again. When I returned to

Australia I was asked to present some memories from Ireland. I contacted Angela. Without prompting she said, 'Of course you'll talk about the woman from Meath.' And in distant years if I were ever to encounter Angela Murphy again walking down O'Connell Street in Dublin or perhaps George Street, Sydney we would stop and no doubt, remember that woman from Meath who spoke to us of a love that was boundless, a union that was indissolvable and who gave us a momentary glimpse into the mystery at the heart of it all (Brennan, 2006).

A personal reflection

To prepare for writing this chapter I decided to engage in an exercise: 'Recapturing Past Resources in a time of Change', suggested by John Kunz in *Transformational Reminiscence* (2007). The exercise is designed to help individuals review their life experiences in a chronological manner. It asks individuals to recall events throughout the life cycle, to identify coping skills, 'intergenerational resources' and 'retrospective wisdom' and to apply these to current situations (pp. 11–16).

I was born in The Netherlands and migrated to Australia with my family as a child of three. For several years we lived in Queensland where I remember walking to school on bare feet and basking in the warmth of the Australian sunshine surrounded by tropical trees and flowers. My parents struggled with the challenge of migration and relocation and suffered many hardships and setbacks. My mother's parents gave up their life in The Hague where they owned a book shop and migrated to Australia with us but they had both died by the time I was 16. My beloved Oma suffered from dementia for several years before her death and my grandfather, a great student of philosophy with an enormous personal library, died following a stroke. My father died of lung cancer when I was 18. He died with many regrets and full of sorrow, leaving my mother a relatively young widow at the age of 51. The lessons gained from our family experiences and perhaps my need to make sense of them led to a decision to become a social worker. I studied philosophy, psychology, and sociology and worked in various fields of health care. In the late 1970s I became involved in the Australian hospice movement and have continued my involvement in palliative care both locally and overseas ever since. For the past ten years I have lived with an auto-immune condition known as Wegener's Granulomatosis. While this rare form of vasculitis can be treated and controlled, there is, as yet, no known cure.

My illness, which has 'flared' three times since diagnosis, has left me with a severe saddle nose deformity and some breathing difficulty. It is a condition which often results in kidney failure and I live with a certain amount of fear that it will get worse as I get older.

Last year my husband was diagnosed with a rare form of oral cancer and is still suffering the after-effects of a brutal yet, as far as we know, effective treatment. In the midst of writing this chapter my elderly mother suffered a 'significant' heart attack and I left my home in Canada to spend three weeks in Australia during her convalescence. Soon after my return she was readmitted to hospital with a second 'small' attack from which she is once again recovering. In coping with all of this I have had to draw on several different resources. Having worked with dying and bereaved people for so many years I already knew that none of us is immune to illness and hardships. Helen Keller (1903: 17) once said, 'The world is full of suffering but also full of the overcoming of it.' I know that all kinds of hardships can be overcome. I already had a lot of knowledge about coping with illness and in some ways, I found it easier to seek and use support. This is not to say that I didn't experience rage, fear, anxiety, and distress or at times doubt my sanity. What the Kunz life review exercise helped me to recognize was how much strength I continue to draw on from my family and cultural heritage, the courage of my ancestors and my experiences as a social worker.

Westwood and McLean (2007: 183) suggest that life review can be a 'therapeutic and beneficial process, fascinating, exciting and freeing all at the same time'. They also remind us that 'opening up of painful memories associated with traumatic events during life review need to be managed appropriately for healing to occur'.

In reviewing my life in this exercise I certainly experienced both the beneficial and the painful aspects. My sense of self has been 'singed by illness' (Broyard, 1992: 6). I am not terminally ill and can only guess at how challenging this kind of life review might be for a person who is in their last weeks or days of life.

Some of the life review and reminiscence literature is disquieting in its enthusiasm and failure to appreciate just how threatening and painful it might be to review one's life at the very end of it. There are signs of a growing industry with a plethora of techniques, kits, and packages and conferences devoted to reminiscence. An emphasis on products such as a book or DVD and facts rather than process may not be as beneficial as the experience of actually being with someone who listens attentively to the life story. For example, The *Self-Discovery Tapestry Kit* developed by Meltzer (2001) is described as a 'colourful interactive life review instrument which will revolutionize reminiscence strategies'. These techniques, products, and bold claims may underestimate the struggle and complexity involved and may even represent the need to defend against the underlying anxiety that close encounters with dying and death arouse. There may be secrets that the teller wishes to remain secret. Not all hurts can be healed or resolved. It is all very well to claim that resolution of old conflicts, forgiveness, declarations of love, and the discovery of meaning are the goals of life review it may not be realistic or possible for many people to achieve such goals. Worse still, the expectation that dying people will complete their unfinished business in this way may add to an already heavy burden of physical unwellness.

Stories represent the very foundation of hospice care. Over the past four decades modern hospice and palliative care services throughout the world have been inspired by the stories of dying patients, their families, and communities. The tools of life review and life story work can be used to bring comfort and meaning to patients and their families at the end of life and during bereavement. Stories may also be used to attract necessary resources for the continuation of services and to provide education and training. Nonetheless, it is important to remember that whatever we learn will only ever be a selective version or a sample of the complexity of a person's life. The best stories as John O'Donohue (2003) reminds us, suggest what they cannot name or describe. He writes:

> A human life is the most complex narrative of all; it has many layers of events which embrace outside behaviour and actions the inner stream of the mind, the underworld of the unconscious the soul, fantasy, dream and imagination. There is no account of a life that can ever mirror or tell all of this. (p. 147)

References

Attwood, M. (2006) *The Tent*. McLelland and Stewart, Toronto.

Bayliss, M. (2007) *Scrapbook Your Life Story and Heal Through the Process: Scrapathy*. Imaginif, Edge Hill.

Birren, J.E., Deutchman, D.E., and DeVries, B. (1995) Method and use of the guided autobiography. In *The Art and Science of Reminiscing* (eds. B. Haight and J. Webster). Taylor and Francis, Washington, DC, pp. 165–77.

Brennan, F. (2006) The woman from County Meath. *Annals of Internal Medicine*. **144**(11), 864.

Broyard, A. (1992) *Intoxicated by my Illness*. Fawcett Columbine, New York.

Butler, R. (2002) *Age, Death and Life Review*. Hospice Foundation of America Teleconference, Living with Grief: Loss in Later Life. Available at: http:www.hospice-foundation.org/teleconference/2002/butler.asp

Erikson, E. (1963) *Childhood and Society* (2nd edn), Norton, New York.

Frank, A. (2002) *At the Will of the Body: Reflections on Illness*. Mariner Books, New York.

Haight, B. (2001) Sharing life stories: acts of intimacy. *Generations*, **25**(2), 90–93.

Irish Hospice Foundation (2006) *Lifestory: A Creative Guide for Recording a Life Story with Contributions from Well Known Irish Writers*. Irish Hospice Foundation, Dublin.

Keller, H. (1903) *Optimism*. Merrymount Press, Boston.

Kleinman, A. (1988) *The Illness Narratives, Suffering, Healing and the Human Condition*. Basic Books, New York.

Kuhl, D. (2002) *What Dying People Want: Practical Wisdom at the End of Life*. Public Affairs, New York.

Kunz, J. (2002) *The Joys and Surprises of Telling your Life Story*. Superior: centre for continuing education/extension. University of Wisconsin-Superior.

Kunz, J. and Soltys, G.F. (2007) *Transformational Reminiscence: Life Story Work*. Springer Publishing Company, New York.

Lester, J. (2005) Life review with the terminally ill-narrative therapies. In *Loss, Change and Bereavement in Palliative Care* (eds. P. Firth, G. Luff, and D. Oliviere). Open University Press, Maidenhead.

Lichter, I. (1993) Biography as therapy. *Palliative Medicine*, 7, 133–37.

Meininger, H. (2006) Narrating, writing, reading: life story work as an aid to (self) advocacy. *British Journal of Learning Disabilities*, **34**(3), 181–88.

McKeown, J., Clarke, A., and Repper, J. (2006) Life story work in health and social care: systematic literature review. *Journal of Advanced Nursing*, **55**(2), 237–47.

Meltzer, P.J. (2001) *The Self-Discovery Tapestry Kit*. Life Course Publishing, Redondo Beach, CA.

Menzies Lyth, I. (1988) *Containing Anxiety in Institutions, Selected Essays*. Free Association Books, London.

Neimeyer, R. (2001) *Meaning Construction and the Experience of Loss*. American Psychological Association, Washington.

O'Donohue, J. (1998) *Anam Cara, A Book of Celtic Wisdom*. HarperCollins, Glasgow.

O'Donohue, J. (2003) *Divine Beauty: The Invisible Embrace*. Bantam Press, London.

Oliviere, D. (2002) Learning in palliative care: stories from and for my journey. In *Journeys into Palliative Care: Roots and Reflections* (ed. C. Mason). Jessica Kingsley, London.

Parkes, C.M. (1972) *Bereavement: Studies of Grief in Adult Life*. Tavistock, London.

Pilotlight (2007) *Dying to Know. Bringing Death to Life*. Hardie Grant Books, Victoria.

Raphael, B. (1984) *The Anatomy of Bereavement*. Basic Books, New York.

Rossouw, R. (2003) Life story Book Work. *Child and Youth Care*, **21**(6), 14–16.

Sheldon, F. (1997) *Psychosocial Palliative Care: Good Practice in the Care of the Dying and Bereaved*. Stanley Thornes, Cheltenham.

Westwood, M. and Mclean, H. B. (2007) Traumatic memories and life review: individual and group approaches. In *Transformational Reminiscence: Life Story Work* (eds. J. Kunz, and G. Soltys). Springer Publishing Company New York, pp. 181–96.

Whiting, P. and Bradley, L. (2007) Artful witnessing of the story: loss in aging adults. *Adultspan Journal*, Fall, **6**(2), 127.

Resources

www.personalhistorians.org
www.reminiscenceandlifereview.org
www.creativeaging.org
www.storycorps.net
www.lifestory.net
www.youtube.com
www.yourlifestory.org
(Source: Kunz and Soltys, 2007)

A Guide for Recalling and Telling your Life Story
Southeast Florida Center on Aging
800-854-3402
www.hospicefoundationofamerica.org

Life Story Work: What it is and what it means: a guide for children and young people.
    British Association of Adoption and Fostering.
My Life Story Book, NSW Department of Community Services.

Chapter 12

The meaning of illness and symptoms

Jonathan Koffman

Pain is the most common and often the most distressing symptom associated with cancer, with a prevalence of over 90% in the more advanced stages of the disease (Solano et al. 2006). Although treatments to manage this symptom have improved in recent decades, some patients still experience severe pain that may be inadequately controlled, and some are reluctant to take treatment. There is growing evidence that those from black and minority ethnic groups have different experiences of pain, often as a result of inadequate treatment or poor access to relevant services (Anderson et al. 2000; Bernabei et al. 1998; Bonham, 2001; Cintron and Morrison, 2006; Cleeland et al. 1997).

Pain and culture

It has been suggested that pain is not just the sole creation of our anatomy and physiology; it emerges at 'the intersection of bodies, minds and cultures' (Morris, 1991). It therefore comes as no surprise that sociologists have long emphasized that ethnicity and culture shape the meaning and interpretation of this symptom, how it is expressed to others, and beliefs about how to live with discomfort or distress (Bendelow and Williams, 1995). There is also some evidence to suggest that cultural beliefs and values serve to create an under-standing that 'normalises' experiences of pain in some groups, which for others may be more problematic. For example, although he is now criticized for crudely reinforcing ethnic stereotypes (Kleinman, 1994), Zborowski attempted to understand and account for differences in the experience and expression of pain among different ethnic groups in the United States. He conducted research in the 1950s and 1960s on pain and its expression among different ethnic groups (Jewish, Italian-Americans, English-Americans, and Irish-Americans) that showed that even within one society, each group had very different norms for understanding their pain and communicating their distress to others. English-Americans and Irish-Americans were stoical, whereas Jewish and Italian-Americans were more vocal about their pain, complaining about their discomfort (Zborowski, 1952; 1969). Zborowski predicted that ethnic differences would diminish through time as successive generations of immigrant descendents came to resemble the host culture.

To date, very little research in the United Kingdom has explored the meanings people with cancer from different ethnic and cultural groups attribute to their cancer pain, despite people from these groups now accounting for 8.1% of the total population, and where increasing numbers are now experiencing advanced diseases. In a recent survey in south London conducted among relatives or close friends of deceased Black Caribbean and White British patients, the former were reported as having more distressing pain, even after adjusting for other demographic, social, and clinical variables (Koffman et al. 2003). The authors suggest that in the absence of other factors, the meanings patients attributed to cancer-related pain may have been shaped by their culture, and are therefore important to explore to understand perceived distress. Meaning has been defined as the nature of the perceived relationships between the individual and his/her social world that is developed within the context of specific events (Fife, 1994). Meanings, which can be shaped by culture, among other factors, have been shown to influence attitudes and responses to illness and its management in the early stage of cancer (Collie and Long, 2005; Wallberg et al. 2003).

The health experience of Black Caribbean people is under-researched, and in many senses this reflects their marginalization in society. The main body of research on Caribbean populations has focused on mental illness (Koffman et al. 1997; Sharpley et al. 2001; Sproston and Nazroo, 2002), heart disease (Chaturvedi and Fuller, 1996; Chaturvedi et al. 1993), and hypotension (Morgan, 1996). Little research has examined the experience of cancer among Black Caribbean people living in the United Kingdom, despite their increasing numbers. In this chapter, I draw upon the experience of conducting a recent narrative-based research study among Black Caribbean and White British patients with advanced cancer to explore how their accounts of cancer pain were shaped by cultural differences. The findings from this research are then translated into practical implications that can inform initiatives to better manage clinical and social care for patients from different ethnic and cultural backgrounds. The study was conducted in three south London boroughs with the highest concentrations (11.4%) of Black Caribbeans in the United Kingdom. Patients were identified by in-patient and community-based palliative care teams and from oncology out-patient and lung clinics.

Conducting the interviews

Narrative research is defined in different ways, depending on the subject of study, the manner in which it is being studied, and the purpose of the study. It has been argued that there is 'no rigid recipe of what counts as a story' (Robinson and Hawpe, 1986: 112). Some definitions are so broad that they include nearly everything. Others are quite limited focusing on one aspect of narratives. Bertaux and Kohli (1984) suggest that narrative-oriented interviewing consist of two distinct parts. First, the interview contains an extensive narration by the participant. During this phase the researchers restrict their involvement to encouraging the continuation of their story. Second, the authors suggest that the researchers actively engage with topics discussed in the narrative, seeking clarification and introducing additional issues that may have been implied or omitted). Researchers also need to be aware of how questions are framed (Chapter 3 provides a further discussion of narrative interview methods).

For this reason the interviews were informal in style and loosely followed a topic guide that was initially guided by a review of the literature and then developed following discussions with a cancer patient advocacy service for the local Black Caribbean community. Interviews began with general questions that asked patients in their own words, and at their own pace, to explain what they understood about cancer and it causation. Questions were framed in such a way that they explored what bothered or troubled them about their illness, particularly as their disease had progressed. Questions also explored how patients managed to live with their illness. Attempts were made to frame the language of the interview in colloquial terms in order to make the interview accessible to participants from the two ethic groups, who tended to be older people.

Narrative-oriented interviewing also involves different ways of listening. This is acknowledged by Bornat in her treatment of interviewing as a social relationship with complex emotions on both side of the microphone (Bornat, 2004). Stanworth states that in order to be open and sensitive to potentially important narratives, researchers should try to suspend their conventional expectations about situations (Stanworth, 2004). Although it may appear to have been counter-intuitive, when I listened to participants' accounts of their advanced cancer, I felt it was important to try and separate myself from the idea that their experience – cancer and their impending death – were the worst things that could happen to them. Although a number of patients clearly regarded their cancer, their pain, and imminent death as catastrophic, there were some participants who viewed their situation against what they considered to be more challenging experiences they had experienced during their life. In addition, there were a number of Black Caribbean patients who welcomed their death as they believed this would connect them more intimately with God. I tried to have an open mind, but I never expected these responses, and they illustrated how easily expectations about illness could have had the potential of preventing me from hearing what participants were actually saying.

Patients' account of their pain

A total of 28 Black Caribbean and 19 White British cancer patients participated in the study; 23 Black Caribbean and 15 White British patients reported that they had experienced pain associated with their cancer. Twenty-four patients offered accounts that governed how they related to their cancer-related pain. Four meanings were evident and helped to understand how patients make sense of their experiences. These meanings are summarized in Box 1.

Pain as a challenge

One view of pain as a challenge represented a task or a hurdle that imposed demands on individuals and that needed to be overcome and mastered by any means available. Four patients (three Black Caribbean and one White British) described their pain in this way. Although Joseph, a 68-year-old Black Caribbean man with prostate cancer described his pain as being '*overwhelming*' and as '*reducing*' him to tears, he nevertheless viewed his pain

Box 1: The meanings of cancer-related pain		
Meaning	**Description**	**Sub-categories**
Pain as a challenge	A task or hurdle that needs to be overcome	Mastering the challenge Unable to meet the challenge
Pain as an enemy	An unfair attack by hostile force	-
Pain as a test of faith	Associated with confirmation of religious belief	Meeting a test of faith Unable to overcome a test of faith
Pain as a punishment	Characterised by theme of wrongdoing	Justified and unjustified punishments

as a challenge that he believed he could successfully negotiate. In order to accomplish this, he talked about setting his own distress in the context of the greater suffering experienced by other cancer patients around him. This comparison enabled him to view his situation more positively. When I asked him to describe his pain he said it was 'horrible':

> It makes me cry. I cried like a man. Especially when you go to lay down. I went to a respite, which is in Brixton. . . . It make a difference to (me) . . . it helps me to realise that there's other people is worse than me and is suffering and is worse than me, so that bring me back to reality.

Both social class (Kelleher, 2002; Williams and Bury, 2002) and gender (Moynihan, 1998) have been recognized as strongly influencing beliefs about illness and reactions to it. Another male respondent who emphasized overcoming the challenge of pain was Bill, a 69-year-old White British man with colon cancer who had at various times in the past engaged in high-risk, demanding occupations, for example, erecting scaffolding and boxing. In his account, Bill trivialized the impact of his pain on his life and exhibited a bravado that may have reflected his up-bringing and male-dominated career in south-east London. He commented:

> I'll take it as it is. (You can) look the world straight in the eye and handle it as it goes. There's no chips on the shoulder, no worries about it. Neither does my family. We'll just carry on. . . . My outlook is much stronger probably than a normal person. And I mean that. . . . The only two things ever I done was fight and hang about with one arm two hundred feet up in the air most of my life. The discipline of the whole thing I've been through. Obviously I'm not dancing up and down and I don't want to die, but I'm er I'm not frightened. Not . . . I'm not er . . . I'm not frightened of it or nothing.

In contrast to the notion of pain as a challenge that could be mastered, five Black Caribbeans and one White British patient, all of whom reported they were in receipt of pain medication, believed that it was quite impossible to rise to their own challenge of mastering their pain. Some of these patients stated they would only be offered a release from distress in their death. This view is illustrated by Merlene, a 68-year-old Black Caribbean woman with stomach cancer:

> I feel sometimes, well . . . what am I living for? I'd better *die*, instead of suffering with all this pain. That's how I feel. . . . Well, when you die, no more pain.

Another Black Caribbean woman called Gwen with stomach cancer remarked that until her pain had been partially relieved by medication, she similarly believed death would have been preferable:

> There were days when the pain was just so intense I would say I'd rather just end it all. I mean, when I went to the operation, I know it's a horrible thing to say, but when I went to the operation I thought if I don't make it off the operating table, it won't be

a great loss to me. I know my children would have to you know, it would be hard for my children, but to me I could cope with death rather than struggling with cancer, which is a horrible thing to say.

Pain as an enemy

Seven patients (four White British and three Black Caribbean) viewed their cancer-related pain experience as 'an enemy'. This characterization of pain referred to situations where respondents described their pain as an unfair attack by a hostile force. Patients' statements categorized in this way were made up of military metaphors, focusing on the need to 'fight' or 'defend' themselves from their pain. Others were more ready to capitulate. This meaning of pain was most prominent among those patients who were still experiencing pain at the time of the interview. An 81-year-old White British woman with pancreatic cancer used the word 'fight' to describe her strategy of adaptation to her constant pain. Jeanie said:

I used to fight the pain as much as possible . . . it's hardened me I think, and that's why I can (now) fight pain off.

In contrast, Reginald, a 78-year-old White British man with prostate cancer was unable to respond to his enemy in these positive terms. He appeared to be very embittered, frustrated, and rendered helpless by his situation, wanting very much to repress his ongoing campaign against his pain. He explained:

(It's) like the War. It's horrible and you want to forget it. But you can't.

While still viewing pain as an enemy, two, White British patients departed from the more common metaphor of the battlefield to convey their experience. Instead, they perceived their pain as a wicked, malevolent, or demonic entity. Freedom from pain could only be achieved through its exorcism. This is illustrated through Becky, a relatively young woman in her thirties with an adenocarcinoma. She believed that when her pain was at its most severe, only through the resection of her stomach – the source of her pain – would she find palpable relief. This would then foster a degree of control back into her life:

I look at it like there's been a devil in me. . . . I wanna curl up and I wanna er . . . some days, you know, I feel like cutting my own stomach and taking it out. It's . . . you have to do something to . . . I, I can't explain it so good.

Pain as a test of faith

Pain represented a trial or test of faith for a small number of Black Caribbean cancer patients. This meaning was associated with confirmation and strengthening of religious belief and loyalty to God. Analysis of this theme revealed two groups: patients who met or successfully overcame their test or those who were overcome by it. Engaging with pain as a test of faith offered two Black Caribbean patients with an opportunity to do something positive in light of the unknown. For example, Alice, a middle-aged Black Caribbean woman was convinced that her breast cancer and her enduring pain represented a test similar to that of Job in the Old Testament. This meaning enabled her to view the world not as an arbitrary place of uncertainty, but one where order and predictability were present even during cancer. She explained:

> In s- some way I think he, he's tested me. . . . To see how strong I am, how strong my faith is, how much I believe in him. I don't know if you ever read about in the Bible about Job and the songs erm, you know, in the Bible, this book, song of Job. . . . And even his wife turned around and said, 'You silly man', or whatever, 'Stupid man. Curse God and all that'. And he's saying to her, he's so, so determined, he said, 'No, woman, you can't be like that. You can't curse God and all that', and he kept his faith. . . . I'll keep hanging on, and I'm hanging on till the last minute.

One Black Caribbean patient, however, had greater difficulty comprehending why he was being tested and therefore was unable to rise to the challenge of attempting to overcome it. The pain he experienced was at times incessant and gave no indication of abating. He represents a modern parallel to Job, attributing his pain to divine intervention. Like Job, this patient exhibited despair and anguish in the manner which he was being tested. His narrative moves on to points of confrontation and bargaining that will terminate his test:

> Sometimes at night time I go to bed and when the pain is so much I turn everywhere in the bed and the pain is the same. I say, 'Why the good Lord keeping me here? Why don't he take me?' Yeah, I've all those feelings. I say, 'Why are you keeping me? Why don't you take me?' Because I'm in pain.

Pain as a punishment

Pain as punishment was characterized by a theme of wrongdoing that justified retribution and distress. This theme was voiced by four Black Caribbean patients who perceived their pain as being justified, or who found no evidence of wrongdoing in their lives to account for their situation and therefore considered their punishment as being unjustified. Of these patients, two believed the source of their pain as a punishment was justified and the distress it caused them emanated from group sin. Although there is no evidence from the interviews that these patients had at any time refused pain relieving medication, they still believed that denying transgression and wrongdoing would obstruct any chance of correction or healing from taking place. This equanimity or accommodation enabled these patients to find meaning and growth through their distress. For example, Franklyn, a 72-year-old with prostate cancer attributed his illness and pain to a justified punishment believing all humankind was guilty of wrongdoing. By departing from God's guidance and taking his love for granted, punishment was a reality people had to share in. He explained:

> Franklyn: I'm making lots of mistakes and want to improve.
>
> JK to Franklyn: How do you think this affects your cancer and the problems you have?
>
> Franklyn: Sin is a little word name 's' 'i' 'n'. I know what it comes from: – disobedience.
>
> JK to Franklyn: Disobedience? If I'm hearing you right, did you have anything to do with it?
>
> Franklyn: . . . When God made this world and put man here, he didn't just put us here and say: 'Alright, just stay and enjoy yourself on me!'

Elston, however, had far greater difficulty understanding the justification for his punishment illustrating that the randomness of disease could be very threatening and upsetting. As he put it:

> Elston: The worst part of it, the cancer, is the pain . . .
>
> JK to Elston: Do you ever ask yourself why this has all happened?
>
> Elston: Many times. Many times.
>
> JK to Elston: What sort of questions go through your mind?
>
> Elston: Why? Why me? Cos I don't deserve this.

Discussion of the study findings

This is the first narrative-based study to explore and compare the meanings of cancer-related pain among Black Caribbean and White British patients in the United Kingdom. While pain was the central feature of the accounts of many patients, irrespective of their ethnic group, the interviews uncovered some interesting differences between Black Caribbean and White British patients' narratives. The first main difference was that more Black Caribbean than White British patients reported that they experienced this symptom, and more of these patients reported refractory pain or pain that was still present at the time of their interview, despite receiving medication.

The second important finding relates to the similarities and differences in the ways that Black Caribbean and White British patients attributed meanings to their pain and expressed it during their interviews. According to Yalom (1980) meaning is created by individuals and is not something that is pre-existing. Among other factors, culture shapes the meanings we bring to the world, and this has relevance in understanding the experience of cancer and cancer-related symptoms that challenge our views of the world as being purposeful and coherent. The study found that both ethnic groups narrated pain as an enemy and pain as a challenge, although more Black Caribbean than White British patients referred to their pain as being a challenge they were unable to meet. There is no suggestion in the data that Black Caribbean patients were denied medication or adequate levels of medication to assist them in their 'fight'. Notions of pain as a test of faith and pain as a punishment were specific to the accounts of patients from Black Caribbean groups, and both appeared to be related to strong religious faith and belief in God.

For those Black Caribbean patients who considered their pain to be a justified punishment, this meaning at first appeared to be contradictory. Patients did not refuse treatment for their pain, yet its presence had fulfilled, or continued to fulfil, important functions; it possessed redemptive qualities and offered a means of getting closer to God. Moreover, instead of being perceived as being maladaptive or negative, justified punishments were perceived by Black Caribbean patients as being a positive and active response to their illness that strengthened character. Research among church-going African-American people with cancer has similarly noted that suffering at the end of life is regarded as noble (Barrett and Heller, 2002; Bolling, 1995; Sullivan, 1995). This position is in stark contrast with Charmaz's (1983) research among a predominantly White American, female patient population with heart disease, cancer, and multiple sclerosis where she noted that 'The language of suffering severely debilitated people spoke was a language of loss. They seldom talked of gaining a heightened consciousness of the world, revelations about self or insight into human nature from their experiences' (p. 91).

A number of meanings of pain observed in this narrative-based study appear to support some aspects of the 'Meanings of Illness' framework developed by Lipowski for conceptualizing how people cope with illness (Lipowski, 1970; 1983). He proposed eight meanings of illness where patients may respond differently to their situation, some viewing it positively, as a challenge, while others negatively, for instance, as a punishment or a form of loss. This framework acknowledges that meanings may be shaped by inter-personal factors such as age, personality, values, and beliefs, the likelihood of cure, and prognosis.

Although Lipowski's framework offered a useful and accessible agenda to assist health care professionals and researchers to both explore and understand the meanings that patients give to their cancer and its associated symptoms (Luker et al. 1996; Barkwell, 1991), this research suggests that its current structure requires redefinition and reinterpretation. First, the interpretation of the meaning of pain as punishment may not apply to the experience of pain resulting from advanced cancer. Lipowski's original notion of this meaning was related to the potential for atonement leading to a sense of new beginning. Further, he reported patients who held this view sometimes displayed personality changes, initiative, and vigour which were lacking before the onset of their illness (Lipowski, 1983). For patients in this study, however, many of whom were in the most advanced stages of cancer, the possibility of full recovery from their illness, and therefore atonement, was not a reality.

Second, Lipowski states that the meanings of illness seemed to be most prevalent in the cultures he developed the framework for (Canada and the United States). Consequently, the meanings and their interpretations may not apply readily to all cultural groups and contexts. Research using Lipowski's framework, when applied to cancer, has taken place principally among White patient populations, where 'challenge' was observed as being the most frequently reported meaning (Barkwell, 1991; Luker et al. 1996). From a clinical perspective, pain as a challenge allows health care professionals to enter into partnership with patients to find the best combination of analgesia or other approaches to optimize pain management. Other meanings, however, may be present and interpreted differently in other cultural groups. For example, the meaning of punishment proposed by Lipowski, less frequently encountered in other studies (Barkwell, 1991; Luker et al. 1996), is viewed as an emotional struggle where a negative outlook is usually present (Caress et al. 2001). Faced with patients who hold this view, health care professionals are urged to assist them through health-promoting dialogue to reappraise their situation and to seek a meaning associated with positive coping (Ramfelt et al. 2002). However, the findings from this study suggest that where pain was interpreted by Black Caribbean patients as a punishment, despite its distressing nature, it was not always perceived negatively. This challenges the notion of a single universally understood interpretation of this meaning.

Implications for patient-centred care

Meanings expressed by patients about their cancer-related symptoms are culturally shaped and patterned. The research reported in this chapter observed that this finding was most prominent in relation to cancer-related pain where some meanings may have appeared to be inappropriate and even anti-therapeutic from what is considered usual (Bendelow and Williams, 1995; Juarez et al. 1999). Participants in this category included Black Caribbean patients who viewed their pain as being a justified punishment. However, this meaning did not represent a negative illness attribution. Further, this meaning attributed to their pain appeared to help them comprehend their experience and successfully accommodate it within their lives.

Research suggests that health care professionals' attitudes frequently dominate patients' responses to their experience of pain (Rogers and Todd, 2000; Watt-Watson et al., 2001). Health care professionals have therefore been criticized for patronizing patients by ignoring their 'illness narratives', or the meanings that govern how they understand and accommodate their illness (Kleinman, 1988). Kleinman's concern therefore supports the sentiment that:

> pain is whatever the experiencing person says it is, and it's as bad as the patient says.
> (McCaffery and Thorpe, 1988: 113)

Importantly, this notion can also be applied to other symptoms. Illness narratives should therefore be viewed by health and social care professionals as an important source of information in the overall process of arriving at a more complete picture of a clinical problem. They are also helpful in understanding and resolving problems around diagnosis, treatment, and care. Box 2 therefore lists some of the questions that health care professionals can use in their work with patients.

Box 2: Patient-centred questions that can be asked when assessing pain and other symptoms

- Why do you think you have this pain?
- What does your pain mean to you?
- How severe is your pain? How long do you think it will last?
- Do you have any fears about your pain? If so, what do you fear most about your pain?
- What are the biggest problems that your pain causes you?
- What kind of treatment do you think you should receive? What results do you hope to receive from the treatment? Do you have any concerns about treatment?
- What cultural remedies have you tried to help you with your pain?
- Who, if anyone, in your family or among your friends do you talk to about your pain? Do you have family and friends who can help you because of your pain? Who helps you and how?
- Do religion and/or spirituality feature within your life? Have they helped you understand why you are in pain? Do they help you live with your pain?

Despite palliative care having already developed an important curriculum to address these issues, the tension between comfort care and the increasing medicalization of the speciality means a number of lessons appear to have been repressed (Clark, 2002). In the early 1960s, Dame Cicely Saunders proposed the concept of 'total pain'. This concept included important patient-centred concerns, for example, psychological, social, emotional, and spiritual dimensions of pain (Saunders, 1964). This approach viewed patients' illness narratives as a key to unlocking other issues and as something requiring multiple interventions for their resolution. 'Total pain' was inextricably tied to narrative and biography, emphasizing the importance of listening to a patient's story with an authentic curiosity to understand their experience of their distress and how it could be managed. More recently, Derek Doyle supported this sentiment when he commented:

> What does it profit a doctor if he can prescribe opioids yet not know how to listen actively to those who need his help and humanity? Palliative medicine and pain control are as much exercises in communication as they are applied pharmacology.
>
> (Doyle, 1989)

References

Anderson, K. O., Mendoza, T. R., Valero, V., Richman, S. P., Russell, C., Hurley, J., DeLeon, C., Washington, P., Palos, G., Payne, R., and Cleeland, C. S. (2000) Minority cancer patients and their providers: pain management attitudes and practice. *Cancer*, **88**, 1929–38.

Barkwell, D. P. (1991) Ascribed meaning: a critical factor in coping and pain attenuation in patients with cancer-related pain. *Journal of Palliative Care*, **7**(3), 5–14.

Barrett, R. K. and Heller, K. S. (2002) Death and dying in the black experience. *Journal of Palliative Medicine*, **5**(5), 793–99.

Bendelow, G. A. and Williams, S. J. (1995) Sociological responses to pain. *Progress in Palliative Care*, **3**(2), 169–74.

Bernabei, R., Gambassi, G., Lapane, K., Landi, F., Gatsonis, C., Dunlop, R., Lipsitz, L., Steel, K., and Mor, V. (1998) Management of pain in elderly patients with cancer. *Journal of the American Medical Association*, **279**, 1877–82.

Bertaux, D. and Kohli, M. (1984) The life story approach. *Annual Review of Sociology*, **10**, 215–37.

Bolling, J. (1995) Guinea across the water: the African-American approach to death and dying. In *A Cross Cultural Look at Death, Dying and Religion* (eds. J. K. Perry and A. S. Ryan). Nelson-Hall Publishers, Chicago, 145–59.

Bonham, V. L. (2001) Race, ethnicity, and pain treatment: striving to understand the causes and solutions to the disparities in pain treatment. *Journal of Law, Medicine and Ethics*, **29**(1), 52–68.

Bornat, J. (2004) Oral history. In *Qualitative Research Practice*, (eds. C. Seale et al.). Sage Publishing, London.

Caress, A. N., Luker, K. A., and Owens, G. (2001) A descriptive study of meaning of illness in chronic renal disease. *Journal of Advanced Nursing*, **33**(6), 716–27.

Charmaz, C. (1983) Loss of self: a fundamental form of suffering in the chronically ill. *Sociology of Health and Illness*, **5**, 168–95.

Chaturvedi, N. and Fuller, J. H. (1996) Ethnic differences in morality from cardiovascular disease in the UK: Do they persist in people with diabetes. *Journal of Epidemiology and Community Health*, **50**, 137–39.

Chaturvedi, N., McKeigue, P. M., and Marmot, M. G. (1993) Resting and ambulatory blood pressure differences in Afro-Caribbeans and Europeans. *Hypertension*, **22**(1), 90–96.

Cintron, A. and Morrison, R. S. (2006) Pain and ethnicity in the United States: a systematic review. *Journal of Palliative Medicine*, **9**(6), 1454–73.

Clark, D. (2002) Between hope and acceptance: the medicalisation of dying. *British Medical Journal*, **324**, 905–07.

Cleeland, C. S., Gonin, R., Baez, L., Loehrer, P., and Pandya, K. J. (1997) Pain and treatment of pain in minority patients with cancer. The Eastern cooperative oncology group minority outpatient pain study. *Annals of Internal Medicine*, **127**(9), 813–16.

Collie, K. and Long, B. C. (2005) Considered 'meaning' in the context of breast cancer. *Journal of Health Psychology*, **10**(6), 843–53.

Doyle, D. (1989) Education in palliative medicine and pain therapy: an overview. In *The Edinburgh Symposium on Pain Control and Medical Education* (ed. R. Twycross). Royal Society of Medicine, London, 165–74.

Fife, B. (1994) The conceptualization of meaning in illness. *Social Science and Medicine*, **38**(2), 309–16.

Juarez, G., Ferrell, B., and Borneman, T. (1999) Cultural considerations in education for cancer pain management. *Journal of Cancer Education*, **14**(3), 168–73.

Kelleher, D. (2002) Coming to terms with diabetes: coping strategies and non-compliance. In *Living with Chronic Illness: The Experience of Patients and Their Families* (eds. R. Anderson and M. Bury). Unwin Hyman, London.

Kleinman, A. (1988) The illness narratives. Suffering, healing, and the human condition. Basic Books, New York.

Kleinman, A. (1994) Pain as human experience: an introduction. In *Pain as Human Experience: An Anthropological Perspective* (eds. M. J. Delvecchio, P. Good, P. Brodwin, B. Good and A. Kleinman). University of California Press, Berkeley. pp. 169–97.

Koffman, J., Fulop, N., Pashley, D., and Coleman, K. (1997) Ethnicity and the use of acute psychiatric beds: findings from a recent census of acute psychiatric patients in North and South Thames regions. *British Journal of Psychiatry*, **171**, 238–41.

Koffman, J., Higginson, I. J., and Donaldson, N. (2003) Symptom severity in advanced cancer, assessed in two ethnic groups by interviews with bereaved family members and friends. *Journal of the Royal Society of Medicine*, **96**(1), 10–16.

Lipowski, Z. J. (1970) Physical illness, the individual and the coping processes. *Psychiatry in Medicine*, **1**, 91–102.

Lipowski, Z. J. (1983) Psychosocial reaction to illness. *Canadian Medical Association Journal*, **128**, 1069–73.

Luker, K. A., Beaver, K., Leinster, S. J., and Owens, R. G. (1996) Meaning in illness for women with breast cancer. *Journal of Advanced Nursing*, **23**, 1194–201.

McCaffery, M. and Thorpe, D. (1988) Differences in perception of pain and the development of adversarial relationships among health care providers. *Advances in Pain Research and Therapy*, 11, 113–22.

Morgan, M. (1996) Perceptions and use of antihypotensive drugs among cultural groups. In *Modern Medicine: Lay Perspectives and Experiences* (eds. S. J. Williams and M. Calnan). UCL Press, London.

Morris, D. (1991) *The Culture of Pain*. University of California Press, Berkeley.

Moynihan, C. (1998) Theories of masculinity. *British Medical Journal*, 317, 1072–75.

Ramfelt, E., Severinsson, E., and Lutzen, K. (2002) Attempting to find meaning in illness to achieve emotional coherence: the experiences of patients with colorectal cancer. *Cancer Nursing*, 25(2), 141–49.

Robinson, J. and Hawpe, L. (1986) Narrative thinking as a heuristic process. In *Narrative Psychology* (ed. T. Sarbin). Praeger, New York.

Rogers, M. S. and Todd, C. J. (2000) The 'right kind' of pain: talking about symptoms in outpatient oncology consultations. *Palliative Medicine*, 14, 299–307.

Saunders, C. (1964) Care of patients suffering from terminal illness at St. Joseph's Hospice, Hackney, London. *Nursing Mirror*, p. vii–x.

Sharpley, M., Hutchinson, G., Murray, R. M., and McKenzie, K. (2001) Understanding the excess of psychosis among the African-Caribbean population in England. *British Journal of Psychiatry*, 178(40), S60–S68.

Solano, J. P., Gomes, B., and Higginson, I. J. (2006) A comparison of symptom prevalence in far advanced cancer, AIDS, heart disease, chronic obstructive pulmonary disease and renal disease. *Journal of Pain and Symptom Management*, 31(1), 58–68.

Sproston, K. and Nazroo, J. (2002) *Ethnic Minority Psychiatric Illness Rates in the Community (EMPIRIC) – Quantitative Report*, HMSO, London.

Stanworth, R. (2004) *Recognising Spiritual Needs in People who are Dying*, Oxford University Press, Oxford.

Sullivan, M. A. (1995) May the circle be unbroken: the African-American experience of death, dying and spirituality. In *A Cross Cultural Look at Death, Dying and Religion*, (eds. J. K. Perry and A. S. Ryan). Nelson-Hall Publishers, Chicago, pp. 160–71.

Wallberg, B., Michelson, H., Nystedt, M., Bolund, C., Degner, L., and Wilking, N. (2003) The meaning of breast cancer. *Acta Oncologica*, 42(1), 30–35.

Watt-Watson, J., Stevens, B., Garfinkel, P., Streiner, D., and Gallop, R. (2001) Relationship between nurses' pain knowledge and pain management outcomes for their postoperative cardiac patients. *Journal of Advanced Nursing*, 36, 535–45.

Williams, S. J. and Bury, M. (2002) Impairment, disability and handicap in chronic respiratory disease. *Social Science and Medicine*, 29, 609–16.

Yalom, I. (1980) *Existential Psychotherapy*, Basic Books, New York.

Zborowski, M. (1952) Culture components in response to pain. *Journal of Social Issues*, 8, 16–30.

Zborowski, M. (1969) *People in Pain*. Josey-Bass, San Francisco.

Chapter 13

Spiritual care and attentiveness to narrative

Rachel Stanworth

According to the novelist Phillip Pullman in his 1996 Carnegie Medal accept-ance speech (Random House Publications, 1996), 'thou shalt not' is very soon forgotten, whereas 'once upon a time' lasts forever. Perhaps this is because narrative and its encompassing cousin, story, combine processes of discovery with those of invention (Ricoeur, 1978: 239). In so doing, they exert powerful influences over both our imagination and our daily lives, even to the point of our dying. My brief here is to consider this potency, its relevance to the spiritual care of terminally ill people, and the qualities required of anyone who wishes to really hear the deeper beat and resonance of another's story; who wishes to understand that stories may be organized as a series of events, but sometimes the sequence 'is only a net whereby to catch something else, the real theme may be, and perhaps usually is, something that has no sequence in it' (Lewis, 1982: 17).

We should also never forget that 'every story someone tells us is a snapshot of their inner world. Stories are symbolic language – a deep communication given in a roundabout way to test the waters of the listener's receptivity' (Longaker, 1997: 146). Nevertheless, in the words of one experienced and respected clinical nurse specialist at the hospice where I work, 'When you're faced with real suffering and you've done everything practical that you can, I sometimes feel communication skills just aren't enough. There has to be something more'. A further aim of this chapter, therefore, is to consider the possibilities for 'anything more' to emerge in our encounters with patients. Specifically, whether there is anything about narrative and story that can provide safe ground when, in shifting and treacherous conditions, it seems there is nothing left in the professional armouries to secure a reliable footing for patients.

Effective palliative care is about helping people to be who they are, literally helping them to become self-possessed, free from the avoidable distractions of physical pain, of social, psychological, and spiritual distress. I hope to make the case that when professionals (and others) learn to become attentive, a free and friendly interpersonal space for patients' stories to emerge is sometimes created. Furthermore, these stories can often have a quality of largesse or 'giftedness' about them, insofar as their potential for healing, as distinct from curing, exceeds anything we might consciously anticipate.

Story's disclosive potential

Story, nervertheless, can wound as much as it can console or inspire (see also Frank, this volume). This is because it has a capacity to show us truths we cannot say or bear to face. Truth may provide a place from which we can start again but 'depth perceptions' about ourselves, and our lives do sometimes hurt and threaten. Story's potency results in large part from the disclosive potential of two of its most powerful tools: metaphor and symbol. When, 'we are speaking about one thing in terms which are seen to be suggestive of another' we are using metaphor (Soskice, 1987: 15). A good metaphor conveys complex thoughts and feelings with impressive economy and is never directly translatable or reducible to literal language. Griffith (2002: 79), reflecting on a counselling encounter, demonstrates the importance of remaining open to this pluri-potential:

'God is like a light', Tracey (Griffith's client) said. 'Yes,' I thought, 'I understand. I know'. But I knew nothing of her light, the light in a doctor's examining room, a light that brings the expectation of pain, a light like a spotlight, one that brings isolating scrutiny. In this realization, I was grateful to all my colleagues who have urged me to inquire about words and metaphors, to value the not-knowing more than the knowing, and grateful to Tracey for releasing me from the confines of my experience.

A further 'interesting thing about metaphor, or at least about some metaphors is that they are used not to re-describe, but to name for the first time ... naming that which has no name'. (Soskice, 1987: 89). I shall never forget, for example, the patient who described himself as 'living on microwave time'. Once removed from the microwave, the last few minutes when a dish is left to stand are crucial. Having recently completed his chemotherapy, I wondered whether there was a sense in which this man, too, was waiting for an outcome. Perhaps, despite his outward passivity, his 'inner world' was active (Stanworth, 2004).

In his *Poetics* (McKeon, 1941) Aristotle argues that metaphor is a sign of genius for it implies an intuitive sense of similarity in 'dissimilars'. It exploits the tension between 'what is' and 'what is not'. For this man, something about terminal illness resonated with his observations of microwave cookery, although the latter is definitely not about dying. Drawing our thinking in unanticipated directions, metaphor thus shows us reality afresh, addressing us at a deep and personal level, often feeling more like an encounter. So why does this matter to the practice of palliative care? Largely because there is growing evidence that professionals tend to shy away from prioritizing patients' stories (Egnew, 2005), and can homogenize patient needs and impose their own fixed expectations (McDermott et al. 2006). Limiting patient storytelling to diagnostic requirements, however, is not entirely incomprehensible. Witnessing another's suffering or regrets is painful. Feelings of powerlessness can compound fears of unleashing overwhelming emotions. Professional reservations possibly reflect a sensed requirement for personal commitment and initiation demanded by such encounters. As many fairy stories remind us, wisdom and insight are often preceded by pain or bewilderment: the needle's prick, choking on an apple, a childhood abandonment. This is why supportive colleagues and teamwork are so important in palliative care. The following statement, however, was made by a participant with learning difficulties at a recent conference on spirituality and health care. He reminds us that sometimes 'There are some things you can only see if you have tears in your eyes'.

If we are to respond sensitively to patients' stories the time has come for palliative care to recognize the potency of symbol. We need a new way of exploring human being-in-the-world' (Heidegger, 1962) which accommodates, not only the empirically true, but all expressions of truth. Derived from the Greek 'symballein', meaning 'to connect', a symbol can embrace any aspect of experience, holding together apparently contradictory features. Consider, for example, the figure of the 'wise fool' or the notion of 'silent music'. Paradox may mark the limits of rationalist vision and knowledge, but we still instinctively recognize its meaning, even when the symbol's point of reference lies beyond scientific enquiry. Just as Moses removed his shoes before the burning bush, or crowds fall silent when Nelson Mandela speaks, we recognize something in the symbolic encounter that speaks deeply and rings true to our experience of being human. The really distinguishing feature of symbol, however, is its grounding in a reality. Thus fire symbolizes hope and protection because it warms and protects but it can also symbolize anger and destruction. This evocation of wide and varying associations makes symbols directly untranslatable, unlocking levels of reality that could not otherwise be apprehended.

Symbolic disclosures by patients thus provide us with 'truths' that may not exist in any freestanding or measurable way, but because they engage our emotions as well as our intellect, they have a potential to change us. They provide, a 'showing that is, at the same time, creating a new mode of being' (Ricoeur, 1976: 88). Thus a movement is always a gesture, and when gesture mediates symbolic meaning, even the gentlest of touches can console where words may fail. It makes sense, therefore, for a patient to describe herself as 'spiritually comforted' because her nurse brought a cool pillowcase when she felt feverish. I wish to argue that this transforming potential reaches even beyond the generally accepted limits of narrative therapy and meaning reconstruction (Neimeyer, 2003), that symbol and metaphor sometimes disclose distant and meaningful horizons.

Life is, however, larger than language, and experience entices us beyond the limits of all our stories. This is especially so at the end of life when the issues we most want to understand are exactly those where either we must speculate or fall silent. Patient anxieties so often expressed in the form of questions such as, 'Why me?', 'Why now?', 'What will happen to me after I die?' are essentially theological, for they point to issues of ultimate meaning and purpose. They express, 'the anxiety of meaninglessness [which] is anxiety about the loss of ultimate concern, of meaning which gives meaning to all meanings' (Tillich, 1962: 47) Interestingly, this move towards theology is less a move towards any concept of God than a return to story:

> The language of theology is the language of symbol. Symbols, whether verbal (as in poem or story) or sensual (as in art or music) have an openness which refuses to tie down that to which they refer, but rather makes it available to individual response and apprehension.
>
> (Polkinghorne, 1988: 194)

In many ways, there is nothing here that is antithetical to the ethos of palliative care which has a stated commitment to personalized and holistic care. Rather, what is being made is the case for an expanded and more inclusive approach which recognizes the contingency and complexity of meaning and its interpretation.

Spirituality

Palliative care has long – and quite rightly – associated spirituality with the human quest for purpose and meaning. However, this approach can be overly reliant upon a model of meaning-making that privileges rational thought and language, neglecting different modes of communication and the experiences of children, of adults with learning disabilities, and others. Similarly, the physical experiences many describe as spiritually significant, occurring in hostile environments (Lane, 1988) or during extreme sports are also excluded (Neitz and Spickard, 1990). Perhaps the excessive familiarity of the two terms has also encouraged a certain sloppiness of thought towards their relative tensions. To achieve one's purpose, for example, one must assume a certain degree of control, but when we experience deep meaning we speak of having been touched or carried away – as per the symbolic encounter. Steindl-Rast (1984: 69) highlights this paradox, which is surely relevant to the poise between 'doing' and 'being' required of good palliative care: 'Unless you take control, you won't achieve your purpose; but unless you give yourself, you can't experience meaning.' Even the simplest act of care embodies these relative dimensions of 'what' and 'how' and very often it is the latter that matters most for, in Dame Cicely Saunders' words, 'the way care is given can reach the most hidden places' (quoted in Kearney, 1996: 2).

Paradox is part of the language of spirit, and spirituality itself does not yield easily to definition. Like the horizon it can never be seized and this can be daunting for both practitioners and for those who are dying. I have found it helpful to regard the term spirituality as referring to the interpretive story and values of shared human experience. It is not necessarily anchored in a religion but is autonomous and free-ranging crossing boundaries of religion and culture. In short, spirituality discloses to us the 'really real' (Geertz, 1973: 125), encompassing the most fundamental and comprehensive account of life and its underlying value. This account, however, is less about making sense *of* events, than the situation where events make sense *in* us, and this may be literally incommunicable.

Certainly, spirituality's combination of human and ultimate meaning is often easier to recognize than it is to explain, relying as it must upon metaphor and symbol to 'say, the unsayable'. There is nothing necessarily complex about this, and elsewhere (Stanworth, 2004: 2) I describe an elderly frail woman who prevented her nurses from clearing the bedside locker of her dead flowers. Upon questioning, she explained that she wanted to keep them because as the petals fell, 'they help me to let go. Although they have left this life, if you look carefully, you can see some are shooting up towards heaven; the ones with seedpods. Those seeds won't grow of course, but the thought is heavenwards.... I do wonder what it's like after you're dead'. The fading blooms suggest beauty in decay, point to the meaningful rhythms of nature, both promising and withholding future life – sustaining the sense of wonder and threshold expressed in the final sentence. The flowers draw attention to aspects of reality that generally tend to be overlooked and by so doing their symbolic disclosures both validate and comfort their observer. Spirituality, like the poet, recruits our imagination. It requires us to notice life: a mote of dust hanging in sunlight; a child's smile.

Good palliative care, by definition, embraces good spiritual care because although the spiritual may be a distinctive dimension of human experience, it is not distinct. It cannot be separated from all that is. There is, however, a further point to be made about this patient's liberating observations. They can be approached in terms of the experience and language of grace (Haight, 1979). In theological thinking the graced experience is not of our own making but breaks gratuitously and unexpectedly into consciousness. At such a moment, regardless of apparently contradicting circumstances, one simply knows there is 'ground beneath one's feet'. Given that its effects, which are always positive, can be detected, yet its cause is inexplicable, the graced experience is thus as much a question as it is an answer. In further paradox, grace is not distinctly perceived as such but comes to people through the concrete and singular circumstances of their lives.

Where grace, spiritual care, and story are concerned, the most anyone can do is to 'prepare for an experience we cannot evoke' (Louth, 1994: 3). This does not let professionals 'off the hook', however. It is still a tall order to combine the highest clinical, and other standards of care, with a quality of presence that speaks of openness and availability. The generally accepted 'Good Death' is a story of resolution, whereas the unpredictability of encounter just outlined may evoke professional frustrations, defensiveness against fears of dying and even expose matters of personal ego – a thwarting of the desire *for me/my team* to make everything right for *my/our* patient, a desire that Das Gupta, Irvine and Spiegel also discuss (Chapter 2).

More positively, however, recognizing the limits of personal responsibility can diffuse some of the pressures involved in care giving. It may sound a platitude but we can only do our best. Some things we are simply unable to 'fix' and it may be inappropriate or even damaging for us to try. Story lines that encourage us to think we can are personally and professionally dangerous. Humility is less about false modesty or despondency than about trust. Specific guidelines on spiritual care, religious or spiritual care practices are still relevant, of course, but our remit ends when patients' can most be themselves and their stories, reflections, dreams, and memories can flourish to do their own work.

Converging interests

The convergence of the existential and the practical in palliative care is perhaps unsurprising. There is, after all, a natural tendency to reach for the comforting narratives of childhood at the end of life. Sadly, if such stories have not accompanied and informed our ageing, they are simply souvenirs. In all likelihood they will be discarded, with emotions ranging from sadness to bitterness, from disillusionment to anger. *In extremis*, any story that is not genuinely one's own will almost inevitably yield disappointment, regardless of whether it is a religious doctrine or the fiction of a loving family. Only by touching and expressing personal meaning in the here and now, by symbolically addressing one's self in a real and meaningful way, is any story genuinely alive. Despite the unpredictability of a story's outcomes, it is this latter capacity that makes it so important in spiritual care at the end of life. A patient may appear to be declining on all fronts, but the disclosures of symbol and metaphor can still convey something of his or her struggle towards self-realization. This potential is still recognizable even when the legitimacy of life's ultimate or spiritual dimension is denounced:

> four givens are particularly relevant to psychotherapy: the inevitability of death for each of us and for those we love; the freedom to make our lives as we will; our ultimate aloneness; and finally the absence of any obvious meaning or sense to life. However grim these givens may seem . . . it is possible to confront the truths of existence and harness their power in the service of personal change and growth.
>
> (Yalom, 1991: 4)

The journey towards personal wholeness, however, is a lifetime's task and from infancy, story provides the metaphors by which we live (Lakoff and Johnson, 1980). Such metaphors mediate all our perceptions, including our experiences of cancer (Sontag, 1978). It is no exaggeration, that when a patient tells us something of his or her life we are being entrusted with their most precious possession: themselves. Given that story creates shared perceptions and common understandings, making us who and what we are, the maxim 'poetically man dwells' (Heidegger, 1976: 131) is not an abstract philosophy. It is an urge instinctive to even the youngest child or the most vulnerable adult. The need for security and safety is lifelong. Nevertheless, as much as story creates 'home' it can also threaten our *status quo* (Crossan, 1975), providing revolutionary, unwelcome, and destabilizing insights.

There was a time when the philosophy of palliative care was a new and unsettling liberation story. There are very many places where it still is. Even where such care is well established, the creation of a space for patients to be themselves, to feel secure and able to say, 'Here I am – and it's alright' is still a good aim. At its most radical level, the desire to know oneself and to be able to say 'I am' is bound up with a search for one's place in the ultimate, and thus spiritual order of things. 'I am here' can be an articulation of spiritual awareness, as well as a plea for acceptance. Interestingly, after their forbidden eating of the tree of knowledge, God did not ask Adam and Eve, 'What have you done?' but 'Where are you?'

Helping a seriously ill person or desperately challenged 'family' to move to a better situation can challenge any skilled and experienced professional. In this sense, home is a metaphor where the concerns of story and of story-making, of spirituality and of good palliative care coalesce. The general point to be made is that:

> If people cannot speak of their affliction they will be destroyed by it, or swallowed up by apathy. It is not important where they find the language or what form it takes. But people's lives actually depend on being able to put their situation into words, or, rather, learning to express themselves, which includes the non-verbal possibilities of

expression. Without the capacity to communicate with others there can be no change. To become speechless, to be totally without relationship, that is death.

(Soelle, 1975: 76)

Through remembering, retelling our stories, or telling them for the first time it is we who are 're-membered'; put back together in a new way, hopefully re-stor(i)ed to a more faithful version of ourselves where 'faith does not require a belief system, and is not necessarily connected to a deity or God, though it doesn't deny one. This faith is not a commodity we either have or don't have, like a musical ability – it is an inner quality that unfolds as we learn to trust our own deepest experience' (Salzberg, 2002: xiv). If, 'suffering ceases to be suffering in some way the moment it finds meaning' (Frankl, 1992), then it is essential for those involved in the care of terminally ill people to pay attention to their stories, to develop a familiarity and ease with the ambivalences, the uncertainty, the emotional range and paradoxes which they will almost certainly contain. Finally, attention to existential issues has been shown to significantly influence patients' quality of life (Mount et al. 2007).

Story and time

Nowhere does story expose more clearly the paradoxes of human existence than when it fractures the carapace of time. Altered circumstances provide new vantage points. As we approach and review the stories of our lives, our past, present, and future mysteriously and mutually inter-mingle, each modulation prompting new and sometimes unanticipated meanings and interpretations. Consider the wife who accidentally learns of her husband's repeated infidelities. In the light of her recent terminal diagnosis, the latest affair may seem relatively inconsequential. What may be devastating, however, is the feeling that her own most precious and intimate memories are now tainted; 'he has stolen my past, made it a lie'.

In contrast, the following thoughts were laboriously one-finger typed by a paralysed woman. During her hospice admission, she moved from being a twice-divorced, conscience-striven Catholic, resentfully dependent on her sister, to a place where she could type:

> I feel free. Before admission I was twisted and knotted about my dependence, my sister's health and her efforts to give me as normal a life as possible. It has been so difficult to let go. My hope is that it [i.e. death] will lead me into peaceful waters. Sailing on a calm sea. I have expended so much anger in the past and have longed to get rid of it. It seems that this tragedy has taken me on that path at last.

What is it that has enabled this shift in attitude, enabled her self-realization against all the odds? Certainly the control of distressing symptoms, her experience of trustworthy nursing and the knowledge that her family was supported were vital. Could, however, this woman's equanimity suggest a deeper healing; an intuited sense of ultimate security – despite all her finite and distressing 'historical circumstances'?

Another important point to be made, alongside noting the unpredictability of reflection for each woman, is that such disparity supports postmodern repudiations of providing a 'final word' on specific events or the human condition generally. Each woman reminds us that life is complex and our articulated grasp of personal and deep issues is often quite limited. In the words of one patient, 'the further you dive the deeper you go'. It can be difficult for professionals who are inculcated in 'evidence-based practice', where evidence equates almost exclusively with observable, measurable 'facts' (see Chapter 4), to appreciate the multiplicity and instability of human experience and meaning; that some truths make themselves felt only by retreating from our grasp; that sometimes what 'works' in spiritual care with this patient, at this time, and in this place, cannot be measured, replicated, or even fully understood.

For each of us and at every stage of life, coming to realize one's own story – in that dual sense of knowing and becoming – presents similar challenges: how do I invent – that is create and discover – a weave of narrative and time to protect me from the cold blasts of the past, yet which still permits me personal integrity? What is it that will most help me to face the present with resilience, yet also realistically, and in my own way? How can I contemplate the future with some hope or faith – in the sense outlined above? These are profound questions and, despite what may be the best of intentions, imposing answers upon a vulnerable listener is nothing less than a violation of personhood. For this reason alone it is vital for anyone working in end-of-life or palliative care to have some grasp of where their own story ends and that of their patient's begins. Facing death is perhaps the most radical of human frontiers and it is hard to envisage helping another without having first learned to live one's own life with some degree of consciousness and attention.

For anyone experiencing a heightened sense of personal finitude there is yet another existential question that may arise, often implicitly. It is the question, 'Am I related to anything infinite?' Interestingly the asking of such a question can also be a form of resistance – an undermining of Yalom's four bleak and questionable 'givens'. Although framed more prosaically, it echoes in the words of this woman shortly after the death of her father: '*He was such a fantastic character, really lovely*', adding wistfully, 'but there have been millions of lovely people with great characters going back through all the centuries and who remembers them now?' This correlation of time and infinity (in the sense of timelessness; not of time going on and on), not only expresses a yearning for unity and wholeness but, paradoxically, through the experience of fragmentation, expresses some intuition of what is actually yearned for.

The answer to her question is felt only because it slips from her grasp. Almost inevitably this argument brings into focus the issue of story's existential purchase. Is it just wishful thinking to detect 'heaven in a wild flower'? (Blake, 1977: 506). Is it a foolishness to try and care for patients in ways that undermine the apparently merciless logic of time? Any conscious and reflective professional who emphasizes the importance of patient narrative, will sooner or later ask just how far does a story go? Is it really possible to speak meaningfully about spirituality and spiritual care?

Mirrors or windows?

For Jung (1965: 171) there is but one all-encompassing enquiry and it is, 'What kind of a story am I in?' If, as has been argued so far, 'language is the house of Being' (Steiner, 1992: 127), is it just a house of mirrors? Are there no windows? Is there no external access either mediated or direct, nor any sense of an approaching 'Other'? Alternatively, do we have access to an 'otherness' with a potential to make us 'other'? These questions matter because they address the ethical dimensions of life. Furthermore, in the stark circumstances faced by many patients, there may be no possibility of re-scripting their life's story that is sufficiently meaningful to salve such feelings as guilt, fear, or shame that are produced by their relationships with other people.

Consider, for example, the patient agonized with remorse because during his military service he was involved in killing innocent civilians. His recollection resonates at the intersection of so many stories: political, personal, ethical, spiritual, and religious. Through counselling or therapy he may acquire helpful insights concerning personal and institutional degrees of responsibility; an understanding of human behaviour under stress, or of the overriding effects of sleep deprivation. He may find consolation in a religious doctrine. This particular man, nevertheless, regarded any such 're-storying' as nothing more than a flimsy justification. None of it brought him sufficient peace of mind and heart to feel, in his own words, 'strong enough to die'.

This is not to argue that such approaches should not be attempted. Very often they are more than adequate to their task, expressing the moral commitment and courage of both patients and professionals. They did not, however, provide this man with a sense of ultimate security. Again it is the postmodern reluctance to cast any final existential verdict on this situation that disallows us from discarding the potential for spiritual care as an irrelevancy. Nevertheless, there can remain 'only the trying. The rest is not our business' (Eliot, 1944).

Returning to the two houses for a moment, however, let us substitute an image strong enough to contain both of their tensions of inner and outer. Imagine story as a raft afloat in a sea of unknowing (Crossan, 1975). The ultimate meaning craved by the man is disclosed only where raft and water meet – at the point that is never 'only water' or 'only raft'. Now there is a place for language to express spiritual concerns, but not in any straightforward descriptive sense. Story thus floats not upon another narrative but upon a silence that relativizes all words. A silence that 'speaks' in the sense of being experienced throughout one's whole being. This is where, despite all contrary evidence one simply knows, 'I am here and it's alright'. This may be rare but it can happen.

Both unpredictable and unattainable through personal effort or technique, such healing is a gift evidenced only by its effects. Why it should be present in one situation, as for the paralysed woman, yet not in another as for the ex-soldier or betrayed wife, is mysterious. Nevertheless, the argument still stands, its audacity supported by those who paint, sew, pray, or meditate to experience an altered sense of time, or those who are inspired by nature, or the wonder induced by a night-sky. The effects of such activities show, although they do not explain, how 'the lyricism of meditative thinking goes right to the fundamental without passing through the art of narrating' (Ricoeur, quoted in Clark, 1990:166).

The critical issue is how do we provide palliative care in this evidence-based age, in ways that do not impede such insights or comfort, that allow patients to explore the limits of their own stories, receiving them in an atmosphere of safety and unknowing acceptance? This contemplative turn may challenge Western ways of sense-making, but it is invitational rather than dogmatic, and seeks to disrupt the perpetuation of a mutual estrangement and distancing. Such estrangement denies that when I kill another I also kill myself. The ex-soldier's suffering could thus be read as an awakening from the illusion of separation, as a paradoxical sign of spiritual growth. For professionals repeatedly witnessing sad or distressing stories, if we allow even the remotest possibility that they may also carry insight and healing, it can be sustaining in the face of apparent hopelessness. The irony is that such awareness, is learned through doing, not through reading. Consequently much of what is written here is necessarily invitational.

Committed attention

Discovery is learning to see the already-present in a new way. The already-present, however, is 'not there' for us until it is seen. Patients' stories are waiting to be heard but we need to listen with a receptivity that goes beyond the mechanistic application of pre-formulated and 'off-the-shelf' communication skills. Important though these are, profound disclosures transcend categorization and technique, they have a quality of gift. We, however, need to be able to receive without our own fears – often an unconscious maintenance of distance by casting patients as 'other' – intervening. If patients' precious stories are not to fall unattended, we should realize (again in the sense of knowing and becoming) an authentic and entirely unsentimental quality of presence that says, 'you are relevant, your life is still relevant. If you want to share I will listen and I will not judge'. This is committed attention (Stanworth, 2002) with its implications of alertness, of readiness and yet also of stillness and of waiting. Bakhtin (1990) writes of the inability to see one's self from every angle, even with a mirror, so that we must ask, 'How do I look? What am I like?' This 'creative witnessing' also has a potential to transform aloneness to wholeness (becoming all-one). Put simply, spending time with my friend makes me feel good. She doesn't have to tell me what a great person I am!

. There is an ancient idea that the eye of the mind sees concepts, the eye of the body sees objects. These are dualistic, whereas the heart sees by entering, by participating in the situation of another on his/her own terms, revealing that he or she is loveable simply because they are. We do not give dignity to another. Rather, when we are attentive we recognize the dignity of the other person and this will be expressed in all our exchanges, regardless of how mundane they are. And so committed attention requires us to accept that acts of care are a summons to ethics, an expression of moral value that can deeply affect another's experience of him or herself.

An attractive paradox operates here because the concept of attention pulls in two directions. It implies a narrowness of focus and concentration to the near at hand. This involves some degree of self-forgetting that can also be refreshing. Who has not lost both themselves and track of time when deeply engrossed? All traditions speak of those who become holy (whole), not by following complex rituals but by being fully present to the near at hand. Such presence requires courage for it implies an openness and commitment to change. Committed attention may be akin to love yet when it is directed towards oneself, it may feel as though it dismembers before it makes whole. It was not for nothing that St. John requested the journeying Dante to show, 'how many are the teeth whereby this love of thine does bite?' (Luke, 1989: 180).

It is thus essential for professionals to continually and responsibly read-dress the questions posed by Vachon and Benor (in Lloyd-Williams, 2003: 176): Where do I concentrate my energies? How are my professional and personal life biased? How often do I put the needs of others before those of myself? How often do I find myself 'doing good' but 'feeling bad'? How do I relieve stress? What do I do for my own healing and renewal? How easy is it for me to ask for and to receive support? What brings meaning and purpose to my life? In short, how may I consciously realize both my professional and my personal life's story?

Certainly, such questions often lead to new and uncomfortable territories. The truly attentive professional remains open to the fact that patients often give or teach us far more than they receive.

References

Aristotle (1941) *Poetics. Introduction to Aristotle*. R. McKeon (ed.), Random House, New York.

Bakhtin, M. (1990) *Art and Answerability*. University of Texas Press, Austin TX.

Blake, W. (1977) 'Auguries of innocence', in *The Complete Poems*. Penguin Classics, London.

Clark, S. H. (1990) *Paul Ricoeur*. Routledge, London.

Crossan, J. D. (1975) *The Dark Interval. Towards a Theology of Story*. Argus Communications, USA.

Egnew, (2005) 'The meaning of healing: transcending suffering'. *Annals of family Medicine*, 3, 255–62.

Eliot, T. S. (1944) *Four Quartets. East Coker*. Faber and Faber, London.

Frankl, V. E. (1992) *Man's Search for Meaning. An Introduction to Logotherapy*. Hodder and Stoughton, London.

Griffith, J. L. and Griffith, M. E. (2002) *Encountering the Sacred in Psychotherapy. How to Talk to People about their Spiritual Lives*. The Guilford Press, London.

Geertz, C. (1973) *The Interpretation of Cultures: Selected Essays*. Basic Books, New York.

Haight, R. (1979) *The Experience and Language of Grace*. Gill and Macmillan, Dublin.

Heidegger, M. (1962) *Being and Time*. Blackwell, Oxford.

Heidegger, M. (1976) *The Piety of Thinking*. London University Press, Bloomington.

Jung, C. G. (1965) *Memories, Dreams and Reflections*. Vintage, New York.

Kearney, M. (1996) *Mortally Wounded. Stories of Soul Pain, Death and Healing*. Marino Books, Dublin.

Lakoff, G. and Johnson, M. (1980) *Metaphors We Live By*. The University of Chicago Press, Chicago and London.

Lane, B. C. (1988) *The Solace of Fierce Landscapes. Exploring Desert and Mountain Spirituality*. Oxford University Press, Oxford.

Lewis, C. S. (1982) *On Stories and Other Essays in Literature*. Harcourt Brace Jovanovitch, San Diego.

Lloyd-Williams, M. (ed.). (2003) *Psychosocial Issues in Palliative Care*. Oxford University Press, Oxford.

Longaker, C. (1997) *Facing Death and Finding Hope. A Guide to the Emotional and Spiritual Care of the Dying*. Century, London.

Louth, A. (1994) *Theology and Spirituality*. SLG Press, Oxford.

Luke, H. (1989) *Dark Wood to White Rose*. Parabola Books, New York.

McDermott, E., Bingley, A. F., Thomas, C., Payne, S., Seymour, J., and Clark, D. (2006) 'View from the observatory. Viewing patient need through professional writings: a systematic "ethnographic" review of palliative care professionals" experiences of caring for people with cancer at the end of life'. *Progress in Palliative Care*, **14**(1), 9–18.

Mount, B. M., Boston, P. H., and Cohen, R. S. (2007) 'Healing connections: on moving from suffering to a sense of well-being'. *Journal of Pain and Symptom Management*, **33**(4), 372–88.

Neimeyer, R. A. (ed.) (2003) *Meaning Reconstruction and the Experience of Loss*. American Psychological Association, Washington, D.C.

Neitz, M. J. and Spickard, J. V. (1990) 'Steps towards a sociology of religious experience: the theories of Mihaly Csikszentmihalyi and Alfred Schutz'. *Sociological Analysis*, **51**(1), 15–33.

Polkinghorne, J. (1988) *Science and Creation. The Search for Understanding*, SPCK.

Pullman, P. (1996) www.randomhouse.com/features/pullman/author/carnegie.html

Ricoeur, P. (1976) *Interpretation Theory: Discourse and the Surplus of Meaning*. The Texas Christian University Press, Fort Worth Texas.

Ricoeur, P, (1978) *The Rule of Metaphor. Multi Disiciplinary Studies of the Creation of Meaning in Language*. Routledge and Kegan Paul, London.

Salzberg, S. (2002) *Faith. Trusting Your Own Deepest Experience*. London: Harper Collins.

Soelle, D. (1975) *Suffering*. Fortress Press, Philadelphia.

Sontag, S. (1978) *Illness as Metaphor*. Penguin Books, London.

Soskice, J. M. (1987) *Metaphor and Religious Language*. Clarendon Paperbacks, Oxford.

Stanworth, R. (2002) 'Attention: a potential vehicle for spiritual care'. *Journal of Palliative Care*, **18**(3), 192–95.

Stanworth, R. (2004) *Recognizing Spiritual Needs in People Who are Dying*. Oxford University Press, Oxford.

Steindl-Rast, D. (1984) Gratefulness, the heart of prayer. *An Approach to Life in Fullness*. Paulist Press, New Jersey.

Steiner, G. (1992) *Heidegger*, Fontana, London.

Tillich, P. (1962) *The Courage to Be*. Collins, London.

Yalom, I. D. (1991) *Love's Executioner and Other Tales of Psychotherapy*. Penguin Books, England.

Chapter 14

Bereavement, children, and families

Patsy Way

This is my story of many stories heard in a small playroom in St Christopher's Hospice in South London where I work in the Candle Project team; a team providing bereavement care to children. Some stories are told of foreign landscapes in countries all over the world. They can also describe internal views of the world, landscapes that have sometimes felt familiar, and sometimes very foreign to me. Together, children and families have included me with generosity in stories that might be exciting and dangerous or flat and hopeless, lonely and heartbreaking, or loving and connecting. Though not foregrounded, inevitably I bring my own traveller's tale into the room as, together, we shape and mould stories in our joint efforts to make sense of the world after a bereavement.

The story you tell about yourself attempts to make sense of events, feelings, and what you have done (Byng-Hall, 1995; Hunt and McHall, 2008). It can help you know what to do next. For bereaved people however, the future is not what it was meant to be. Frank (1995: 53) says that 'Stories have to repair the damage that the illness has done to the ill person's sense of where she is in life and where she may be going' and I would argue that the same is true for children and other family members when bereaved. A death may have been sudden or expected to a greater or lesser degree, but it is a punctuation that can radically change so many things in children's lives. Therapeutic work with stories and narrative can help to make sense of attendant chaos.

I hope here to outline some of my developing thoughts about how I interpret and work with children's narratives and stories, introducing you to Patrick as he challenges 'Mr Trouble'; Shiv searching for teenage identity; Gemma and the 'wicked stepmother' story; and little Jude and Ali who did not have memories of their dead fathers. I will use case-study examples to provide practical insights into how stories can aid therapeutic work with children of different ages. All the names used for children and family members in this chapter are pseudonyms.

My working context

The children and families that I work with attend the Candle Project in St Christopher's Hospice. The project supports children and young people affected by a significant bereavement. Children are seen individually or with their families and parents, and children can also be offered group-based support. I will often, though not always, meet the family, it is not solely the child who is the focus of the referral. This can provide families with a context and can allay concerns that one child in the family has either been 'chosen' or has been identified as having a problem that needs professional intervention. A first family meeting, which might include children of any age, allows a joint telling of the story but does not preclude individual sessions later.

Story-making with children and families

My training is primarily in systemic family therapy in which families are seen as being the 'experts' on their lives; my expertise is in being perhaps a little more familiar and comfortable with conversations that others might find odd, strange, or difficult (Anderson and Goolishan, 1992; Smith, 1997). As I am not part of the family I can perhaps be curious or question areas that are seen as too difficult or unsuitable for family discussion. Sometimes family beliefs and ideas can be so familiar that they go unquestioned. My focus is on trying to understand the unique meanings of stories, within their biographical and social contexts, as well as attending to the meanings created in the family and with me.

I conceive family stories as created in a specific time, place, and circumstance. Just as historically the bards made stories their own and knew that no tale could be told in just the same way twice, every telling is unique. I will make every attempt to 'decenter' (Wilson, 2007: 65–9) myself, as the focus of the telling is on the child or family, although I also recognize that every aspect of myself and my identity (such as my age, gender, and ethnicity) will have an impact on how the invitation to tell the story is understood and on what parts of a story are chosen or left out (Anderson and Goolishan, 1992; Rober, 2005a).

Using Appreciative Enquiry[1] (Cooperrider and Whitney, 2005) techniques, I hope to offer a space in which the story can be told in a helpful way (Appreciative Enquiry is also discussed in Chapter 7). In my understanding of how narratives and stories are produced and take shape, knowledge is assumed to be socially constructed and there are many valid and diverse ways of understanding ourselves and others: 'Individuals construct past events and actions in personal narratives to claim identities and construct lives' (Riessman, 1993: 2).

These ideas can be seen in a multilayered context in which 'we focus on the social context in which the words are spoken' (Rober, 2005b: 4) and the story told. This shifts the focus from notions of objectivity and certainty towards intersubjectivity and therapeutic curiosity.

Thus, even when talking to just one member of the family, one can listen for 'backstories' of family, school, workplace, and community group. This inevitably frames the choices of possible directions in which the conversation may develop. Over time the story will be edited and changed and Kraus (2005) has identified the need for some children to revisit bereavement counselling in updating their story.

So this is my story of many stories. As with all stories it is edited, selective, and would be different if I were to write it yesterday or tomorrow. I hope it creates a dialogue with other chapters in this book about the nature and effect of narrative and stories, use of creative techniques in story-making (Freeman et al. 1997; Gersie, 1991; Roberts, 1994; Sunderland, 2000) and ethical issues in the stance taken in eliciting stories.

Taking children and young people seriously

I am often astonished at how little account is taken of children. For a long time there has been little training in working psychotherapeutically with children, though this is changing and more recently the Child Bereavement Network has greatly raised the profile of the needs of bereaved children. In the wider world, the United Nations has identified universal rights of children (1959) and in the United Kingdom the last decade has seen much focus on the protection of vulnerable children (Brown and Seden, 2003), bullying in schools (Bullying UK and Kidscape) and the contexts and concerns about the safety of children in the community. All of these initiatives give focus to particular qualities of childhood and children, as well children's specific needs for support.

Alongside such developments, however, there are also social discourses that position children as being incomplete, inadequate, and not yet fully formed adults – beings who lack certain capacities. In terms of children's narratives of bereavement, such deficit descriptions are often in evidence in categorizing young children as not having the necessary cognitive abilities and concepts to understand the necessity, inevitability, irreversibility, and finality of death (Kane, 1979; Kenyon, 2001). From this sometimes follows notions that there is little point in explaining death to young children: they will not be affected by the death of someone close to them because they are unable to understand the concept of death.

Further, I would argue that many of the discourses concerning children and power are formed in a climate of fear and justification around safeguarding children.

While of course these are vital conversations for practitioners, they can also narrow thinking and discussion that might help children in other ways. Children will sometimes be silent and say that they 'don't know' when unclear about what they can say and to whom. They are perhaps wisely wary of how information will be used. Perhaps we need to develop thinking more broadly about how adults can use and abuse power in conversations.

Why talk to children? Why talk with the family together?

Wilson (1998) has discussed reasons for choosing to work with children despite the pain and messiness that some adults find difficult in such therapeutic encounters. Talking directly to children often brings surprises and new information to other members of the family. Sometimes different versions or aspects of a story are held by different family members and often children are excluded from key elements, without which the story is confusing. All too often, conversations are closed down in families, and can be completely silenced by death and bereavement. Someone from outside the family may have the mandate, from a position of ignorance, to ask questions that children feel are off-limits. Many families who might describe themselves as open may appreciate support to find a way to talk together about some stories. Sometimes, when difficulties emerge in a family following bereavement a child is designated as the sole problem-bearer and a wider conversation may be able to challenge this view. For example, initial descriptions of Patrick were of a very aggressive child. This denied and obscured the rage later described by other family members following their bereavement and the family story initially focused on Patrick as the problem.

What do stories do?

Sometimes gathering the family together can bring with it the possibilities of new information. However, stories have power and can be dangerous as well as helpful (see Frank, this volume). They have the power to heal or destroy (see Frank, 1995: 54–5). They have a performative function (Eva and Paley, 2006), being selected for a particular audience at a particular time. They can make deep connections with stories well known or shared in a culture. For example, modern children's classics such as Pullman's trilogy 'His Dark Materials', Jacqueline Wilson's 'The Cat Mummy', Tolkein's 'Lord of the Rings', Dr Who and Harry Potter all explore themes of death and loss. Stories can introduce a multiplicity of themes and connections as everyone will hear a story differently and pick up on different aspects and ideas. They can be hugely playful, imaginative, frightening, and educative, widening our horizons using many techniques and media. They can also give shape, substance, and coherence to our memories to link past, present, and future.

What can stories do?

Patrick challenges Mr Trouble

White and Epston (1990), working in systemic narrative frameworks, developed immensely practical and playful techniques which have been used with adults, couples and children (Freeman et al. 1997). In talking about a problem which is focused on an individual they invite joint efforts with people in the wider system to notice the oppressive effects of the problem on a person's life and jointly support them in changing behaviours causing concern. This shifts the focus of blame from one individual towards a united effort to pursue a different, identified and recognized solution. When children are showing behaviours that attract blame and anger from home and school this can be extremely useful.

Mary's voice sounded full of worry and anxiety on the phone. Seven-year-old Patrick had always done well in his primary school but since his father's death teachers complained that Patrick was inattentive, shouted out in class, and was increasingly aggressive with other children. At home he was rude and defiant. His mother was now working full time to keep up mortgage payments and she was tired and stressed. She had endured the agony of watching her husband die of cancer, with all the attendant major disruption to every aspect of their lives. Friends tried to support her but most of her family were in Ireland. Why did Patrick choose this of all times to be so difficult? The final straw was that he had nightmares and woke terrified, needing comforting to settle again. Mary could barely function the next morning at work.

Patrick told the story of his father's illness using the Playmobile figures. He demonstrated in action the distress of waiting for news of his father's death and guessing that daddy was dead after a rushed trip to hospital in the middle of the night. His father had been ill at home and in hospital for a long time. Patrick described the loneliness of wondering what heaven might be like as he lay awake in bed at night, hearing his mother sobbing quietly.

Engaging with him in this, Mary was astonished at the details Patrick had absorbed about the death and funeral and she was able to correct some of his misunderstandings. Patrick had witnessed some medical interventions that had been painful for his father and frightening for him. A consultant from St Christopher's Hospice explained what the doctors had done to try to cure and then to alleviate the distressing effects of the cancer. Patrick began to have a fuller story of events, from different perspectives.

However, Mary was very frustrated that Patrick wanted, as she saw it, to sabotage her efforts to create a new life for them. At school he knew he should 'tell the teacher' when in difficulties with other children but this discourse seemed to be overridden by others in his head and his fists lashed out, followed by trouble and detentions. Trouble was a constant theme with Patrick and his mother. He was happy to draw a character he called 'Mr Trouble' and we began to map together, with Mary's help, his appearances in Patrick's life. Was Mr Trouble more likely to visit at home or school? When Patrick was hungry or not? When it was a special day to do with daddy, such as his birthday or Father's Day? Who was most likely to be around when he came? Who was never around? We learned, for instance, that this never happened when Mrs Jones, his favourite teaching assistant was there. Gradually, we built up a picture of Mr Trouble's habits and the tricks he was most likely to try to get Patrick into trouble. We noticed all the distressing effects on Patrick's life. We also began to plot when 'Mr T' was *not* successful; the times Patrick cleverly escaped an invitation to Trouble, so cleverly that even he was barely aware of it.

It began to occur to Mary how her husband had been the voice of discipline in the family. Patrick explained that Trouble hardly had a chance then because dad made jokes and Anger and Frustration just fizzled. This was a different story for Mary and a revelation to her. Mary recruited Mrs Jones as an ally in noticing trouble in school and together we worked on identifying strategies to manage trouble both at home and school.

I was still concerned about the nightmares that were causing a lot of anguish and disruption. Patrick recognized and drew a new character, Nigel the Nightmare who was on Mr Trouble's payroll. Mary and Patrick tracked his influence on their lives and recorded his visits. I role-played the Nigel character and Patrick rehearsed how he would deal with him when he came in the night. Patrick imagined what advice his father would give in dealing with Nigel (White, 1988) and Mary put a photo of his father by Patrick's bed to remind and encourage him. In less than a month Nigel more or less gave up. He still makes a very occasional appearance but is not taken nearly so seriously.

In this way, a narrative externalizing technique identified a dominant story which focused blame on Patrick in most areas of his life and which he found difficult to escape from following his father's death. Identifying exceptions and inviting family, and school staff to notice and encourage different behaviours changed the story and allowed different capabilities to emerge in Patrick.

What can stories do?

Widen the possibilities in your life: Shiv in search of identity

Hermeneutic, dialogic narrative approaches (see Rober, 2005b) take a different position from externalizing narrative approaches in relation to stories presenting difficulties for individuals. With Patrick, the intention was to change and re-route the story outcome to one that might be more helpful. Dialogic approaches aim to call forth a multiplicity of different and alternative narratives (Bakhtin, 1986) with the idea that different 'voices' or narratives can be called forth in different relationships and situations. It is not a case of selecting either one story or another. When people feel stuck and unhappy multiple stories can be explored to find different responses that might prove more useful, extending family conversations into new, unchartered territories (Smith, 1997).

I was talking to 16-year-old Shiv following the death of his father. The family had migrated from India, and the three children had known the constraints of a very traditional family life there and the difficulties of establishing a new life in England. Shiv's father had been violent and physically abusive, and when he developed a brain tumour, it exacerbated the chaos in their lives. Shiv was still suffering flashbacks nearly a year after his father's death. He was complaining of the anger that arose in him unexpectedly and his reactions created situations that surprised and frightened him, in which he saw himself 'over-reacting to the slightest thing'.

In a previous meeting with his family he had remained fairly quiet as his family described him as lazy and passive and not involved with schoolwork. They thought he was not working hard towards achieving success in the world that would enable him to have a good job and support himself and his mother financially and in other ways in the future.

Shiv told me the same sort of things about his laziness and inattention at school when we met on our own. I could have chosen to explore in detail the effect of Laziness on his school and home life, as with Patrick, using externalizing techniques (White, 1989; 2007). I could have invited him to notice times when he did not allow himself to be invited by Laziness into reacting in ways that he described as unhelpful to himself and others. However, my sense was that, beyond the difficulties created by Laziness in his life, Shiv was being silenced by family stories that were hugely powerful. He was the only boy in the family and unspoken but very negative comparisons with his father were being made by him and his family. I surmised that judgments were being made about how he was similar to this father who did not contribute to the family income and had had longstanding mental and physical health problems. With such a dominant narrative in his head and the fears Shiv had that this would all become a reality in the future, he described how he found it difficult to concentrate in school and how computer games soothed and calmed him, distracting him from flashbacks and some horrific memories of events when his father was alive.

Shiv described ways that physically, emotionally, and psychologically the chaos created in the home by a violent father and the months leading up to his death absorbed a lot of his thinking and energies. Indeed, it would be hard to imagine how it could not. When asked to describe what was 'in his head' he drew a picture, depicting different areas of experience in his life (see Fig. 14.1).

On questioning Shiv and – with his permission, his family and teachers – more closely about the description of laziness and inattention in class, different stories emerged. Some, (not all) teachers had noticed some drop in Shiv's performance since his father's death. However, they also said that Shiv's academic performance could be variable. One teacher noticed an outstanding effort in an exam after a rather average performance in class. Stories emerged of difference and variability, not total negligence and inattention.

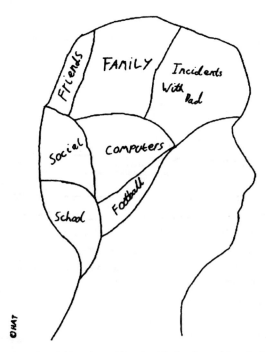

Fig. 14.1 Inside Shiv's head (drawing of head with dominant ideas inside shown).

As we opened up these stories, multiple descriptions emerged of Shiv as protective of his sisters and mother, brave, caring, loving and wily. As a young child he supported his mother and sisters in surviving some terrifying and harrowing situations. Shiv began to widen his descriptions of himself beyond lazy and inattentive. He began to notice when it was easier and harder to concentrate and, though difficult at first, began to talk about wider horizons for his future.

These stories were taken back into a joint family conversation and his mother and sisters began to notice and comment on differences in their perceptions of him. They also began to notice changes in themselves. We used the 'rough rocks' (Stokes, 2004: 162), an exercise using a smooth, a jagged, and a polished stone to represent different memories or feelings about someone who has died. The family used the stones to connect with and share warm memories of their father and also some very difficult ones. All the siblings talked about ways in which they would like to identify with and be like their father (his playfulness sometimes when sober, his generosity of spirit) and also ways in which they would want to be different from him and find different ways in life.

What can stories do? Allow different ways of remembering the past and moving into the present and future

Princess Gemma and the Wicked Stepmother: a story-in-a-story

Gemma's feedback, aged ten, at the end of five sessions with different members of her family at different times, was that bereavement counselling had been 'different from what I expected'. She had thought that it would involve 'going over old ground' and retelling her story in the same way, which was hard. Indeed, she presented as a very bright and articulate girl, with many very difficult memories of living with a very creative and able mother whose behaviour would change when drunk.

Gemma's mother was becoming increasingly ill with alcohol-related conditions which were further complicated by a diagnosis of breast cancer. Gemma told of how, even when quite young, she would try to prevent her mother drinking and would pour the contents of a bottle of whisky down the sink. Many times she had described herself dealing with situations that would daunt most adults. There were less-developed themes in her stories, seemingly more difficult to talk about. She loved her father and his new partner dearly but I also sensed a range of very mixed feelings about the relationship and her loyalties to her dead mother. It led me to start thinking of the descriptions of maleficent stepmothers in fairy stories. Gemma's story focused on the past and on difficult connections to her mother. I wondered if these stories would absorb her and take away energy from future plans. Anderson (Anderson et al. 1986) has argued that 'problem saturated conversations' in families can add strength to entrenched difficulties.

Gemma's story focused on her lone fight with the demons driving her mother to acting in ever-more destructive ways. I wanted to open this up more to allow the family more voice and invite them into thinking with Gemma about the future, without diminishing the harsh realities of the past.

Well-known films, stories, and traditional tales can tap into important family stories and make connections for people on many levels. They need little or no explanation to offer a short cut to cultural ideas and discourses.

I chose the Sleeping Beauty story and customized it in a humorous way to bring out some of the family story, emphasizing the fairy godmothers' gifts to 'Princess Gemma' of Intellignce, Creativity, Beauty, Courage, Wisdom, and Insight. I left gaps in the story for multiple choice options, creating the book in a way that the reader could fill in a preferred phrase at different points in the story. I left the ending open with an invitation to imagine further possibilities. Here is an excerpt from the story:

> Then one day a terrible thing happened, in fact the thing the princess had been dreading. The princess knew that one day the Bottle and the Tumour would kill the queen but she never expected it to be so soon.
>
> It was a truly awful time, beyond the words of a humble storyteller to describe. The queen was dead and the princess was so mixed up because she felt..
> (Choice of the following phrases)
> . . .sad beyond words
> . . .angry
> . . .relieved
> . . .worried
> . . .guilty
>
> The king had managed to keep on running the country in all these difficult times. He had married the Countess Clara. This of course gave her a new title – stepmother to Princess Gemma.
> We all know what kind of press stepmothers have had in Cinderella, Hansel and Gretel etc.
>
> Princess Gemma was thus faced with more confusion because her stepmother seemed to be:
> (Choice of the following phrases)
> . . .beautiful, loving, and caring
> . . .the person Princess Gemma would herself have chosen for the king (based on her own Wisdom, Knowledge, and Insight, given by the fairies)
> . . .difficult and mean and laying down the sort of rules all teenagers hate (in fairness, probably less than many mums and step mums. . .)
> . . .someone Princess Gemma had to share the king's affection with

And, dear reader, ALL this happened before the princess reached Year six!
(and it is more than many many people live through in a whole lifetime)

And now I expect you are waiting for the Happy Ever After bit?
Well unfortunately, for real princesses, it's usually a bit more complicated than that. Plus she's coming up to being a teenager with all those hormones and boys and all that stuff.

And, get real, even without any of this, EVERYONE has worries and homework and bad days and. . .

Well the king and the princess's new stepmother showed how they loved Princess Gemma very, very, much in their different ways.

The princess is growing every day in all those talents and abilities given her by the first six Fairy Godmothers, namely:
– beauty and a lovely smile
– a wicked sense of humour
– intelligence and friendliness
– practical good sense
– creativity, imagination, and happiness
– healthy, stubbornness, and resistance

. . .and the Princess has all these resources to draw on in creating her future.

(Within the story structure, the 'king' (her father) and his new partner ('Countess Clara') and 'Princess Gemma' were invited to add their ideas about her strengths).

This of course is not the end of the story. . .
… … …the princess is just beginning.

This format seemed to me to allow for humour and fun even in talking about some very difficult issues and without diminishing many emotions expressed and experienced in the room. The story was a catalyst in creating a different kind of conversation that surprised Gemma because it did not focus solely on the past but took account of her present and her abilities and support network with which she moves into her future. Using a traditional tale as a framework allowed different thinking and possibilities for Gemma. The family could re-story the events of the past in a very different frame and take up different aspects of the story. The 'multiple choice' format invited ideas of multiple possibilities in thinking about events at different times, and the idea that a story can change and move on.

What can stories do? Co-remembering with very young children

Jude and Ali filling the gaps in the story of daddy

Jude had just been conceived when his father received his cancer diagnosis. His mother lived through a whirlwind in the months that followed, giving birth, nursing a baby at her breast and a very ill husband in bed, and then shortly afterwards organizing a funeral. Jude has no memories of his father in the way we usually think of them. The family used to tell him that dad was on the moon and every night he said goodnight to his daddy while looking up in the sky. A quiet child, he did not make many comments or ask questions about his father. One day, when he was five, with a passionate interest in space travel, he saw a television programme informing him that missions to the moon and far beyond might be quite possible in the future. He immediately asked his mother to book a flight.

Ali was only months old when his father died. His mother had not talked to him about it, thinking that since he had no memories of his father there was no point. She found it too difficult to explain and in any case he would not understand. When he started school however, school staff approached her when he was making strange remarks about his father being dead.

Both mothers contacted the Candle Project feeling concerned that their children needed explanations but not knowing how this could be done since they had no 'real' memories of their respective fathers. Received wisdom among professionals has also often been that since young children do not have a cognitive understanding of the nature, irreversibility and finality of death, there is little point in pursuing this. This view, drawing on a deficit model of children lacking cognitive abilities, ignores other sensitivities and levels of sophistication that even young babies can demonstrate when those around them are grieving (Silverman, 2000).[2]

During a group day, in which these boys were invited with their parents to the Candle Project, they played out, using toys, the events before and after the deaths of their fathers. With their mothers, they talked about how life was at home when dad was there, washing up, going to work and looking forward to the birth. With staff from St Christopher's, and through playing with a toy ambulance and stethoscopes, and other equipment, they understood how doctors and nurses had tried so hard to help their fathers survive. They learned about what it meant to be dead; that your body cannot work anymore and how their fathers were cremated and their ashes collected.

Along the way, weaving into these stories were tales of how proud their fathers had been when they were born, their hopes for them and the ways they had loved and cared for them in the short time they had. Other stories began to emerge of their fathers in the past and the boys were able to ask many questions, then and subsequently. Together a kind of memory of the dead parents was co-created. Arguably these boys have as much right to know and share in such memories as other, older family members with memories of being physically present at a past event. Having the chance to begin to make sense of family stories of their fathers, to begin to imagine them and connect photos, objects, and family stories into a more coherent story, provides a basis for ongoing inclusion when the family are talking about their fathers.

Conclusion

So this is my story of many stories. In Patrick's tale he showed courage in the face of Trouble and when his mother and teacher joined him in looking for exceptions to the story of Patrick being always in trouble, new stories about his behaviour emerged and developed when we played with narrative therapy techniques. With Shiv we evolved a conversation that invited a multiplicity of 'quieter', less-rehearsed stories of his abilities to come to the fore for him to notice and act into, making it possible to question the dominant family story of his lazy disinterest. A traditional fairy story was adapted for Gemma to invite her and her family to view her past and future differently by introducing some lightness, fun, and creativity to generate different possibilities. Finally, with the little boys we were working against the idea that there is no story for children who were 'too young' to have memories when a significant person died and that therefore it is not useful to talk about that person with them.

Different therapeutic story and narrative forms can allow twists and alternative possibilities in real lives, twists and possibilities that it might be hard to think about and reach in other ways. Stories can act and do things (Paley and Frank, this volume) to edit events in ways that help us go on after loss and bereavement.

Notes

1. Used in a variety of contexts including therapy and business management. A practice of asking questions that strengthen a system's capacity to appreciate, understand and heighten positive potential with a focus on discovery and imagination.
2. The Leeds Animation Workshop group offer a DVD outlining simply and clearly the issues for very young bereaved children.

References

Anderson, H., Goolishan, H., and Windermand, L. (1986) Problem determined systems: towards transformation in family therapy. *Journal of Strategic and Systemic Therapies*, 5(4), 1–13.

Anderson, H. and Goolishan, H. (1992) The client is the expert: a not-knowing approach to therapy. In *Therapy as Social Construction* (eds. S. McNamee and K. J. Gergen). Sage, London, pp. 30–38.

Bakhtin, M. (1986) *Speech Genres and Other Late Essays*. University of Texas Press, Austin, Texas.

Byng-Hall, J. (1995) *Rewriting Family Scripts: Improvisation and Systems Change.* Guilford Press, New York.

Brown, H. and Seden, J. (2003) Managing to protect. In *Managing Care in Practice* (eds. J. Seden and J. Reynolds). Routledge and Open University, Milton Keynes. pp. 219–48.

Bullying UK. Available at: http://www.bullying.co.uk (Accessed 01.06.08).

Cooperrider, D. L. and Whitney, D. (2005) *Appreciative Enquiry: A Positive Revolution in Change.* Berrett-Koehker, San Francisco.

Eva, G. and Paley, J. (2006) Stories in Palliative Care. *Progress in Palliative Care,* **14**(4), 155–64.

Frank, A. W. (1995) *The Wounded Storyteller: Body, Illness and Ethics.* University of Chicago Press, Chicago and London.

Freeman, J., Epston, D., and Lobovits, D. (1997) *Playful Approaches to Serious Problems: Narrative Therapy with Children and Their Families.* Norton, New York and London.

Gersie, A. (1991) *Storymaking in Bereavement: Dragons Fight in the Meadow.* Jessica Kingsley, London.

Hunt, N. and McHall, S. (2008) Memory and meaning: individual and social aspects of memory narratives. *Journal of Loss and Trauma* **13**(1), 42–58.

Kane, B. (1979) Children's concepts of death. *The Journal of Genetic Psychology,* **134**, 141–53.

Kenyon, B. L. (2001) Current research on children's conceptions of death: a critical review. *Omega: Journal of Death and Dying,* **43**(1), 63–91.

Kidscape. Available at: www.kidscape.org.uk. (Accessed 01.06.08).

Kraus, F. (2005) The Extended Warranty. In *Brief Interventions with Bereaved Children* (eds. B. Monroe and F. Kraus). Oxford University Press, Oxford. pp. 113–124.

Leeds Animation workshop (2005) *Not Too Young to Grieve.* (DVD, VHS) Leeds, UK.

Riessman, C. K. (1993) *Narrative Analysis.* Sage, London and New Delhi.

Rober, P. (2005a) Family therapy as a dialogue of living persons: a perspective inspired by Bakhtin, Voloshinov and Shotter. *Journal of Marital and Family Therapy.* **31**(4), 385–97.

Rober, P. (2005b) The therapist's self in dialogical family therapy. Some ideas about not-knowing and the therapist's inner conversation. *Family Process.* Dec 2005. **44**(4), 477–95.

Roberts, J. (1994) *Tales and Transformations: Stories in Families and Family Therapy.* Norton, New York.

Silverman, P. (2000) *Never Too Young to Know: Death in Children's Lives.* Oxford University Press, New York.

Smith, C. (1997) Comparing traditional therapies with narrative approaches. Introduction in *Narrative Therapies with Children and Adolescents* (eds. C. Smith and D. Nylund). Guilford Press, New York and London.

Stokes, J. (2004) *Then, Now and Always: Supporting Children As They Journey Through Grief: A Guide For Practitioners.* Winston's Wish, Cheltenham, UK.

Sunderland, M. (2000) *Using Storytelling as a Therapeutic Tool with Children.* Winslow Press, Biscester.

United Nations (1959) Declaration of the rights of the child. General Assembly Resolution 1396 (xiv). Office of High Commission for Human Rights.

White, M. (1988) *Saying Hullo Again: The Incorporation of the Lost Relationship.* Dulwich Centre Newsletter 7–11. Adelaide, Australia. Dulwich Centre Publications.

White, M. (1989) The Externalising of the problem and re-authoring of lives and relationships. Dulwich Centre Newsletter, 3–20. Dulwich Centre Publications, Adeleide, Australia.

White, M. and Epston, D. (1990) *Narrative Means to Therapeutic Ends.* WW Norton, New York and London.

White, M. (2007) *Maps of Narrative Practice.* Norton, New York and London.

Wilson, J. (1998) *Child-focused Practice: A Collaborative Systemic Approach.* Karnac, London.

Wilson, J. (2007) *The Performance of Practice: Enhancing the Repertoire of Therapy with Children and Families.* Karnac, London.

Afterword

William Alwyn Lishman

Narrative, like bread, is the staff of life for most of us. It can inform, illuminate, entertain, and bring relief to both the giver and the receiver. In times of mental stress it often emerges as the high road to regaining equilibrium. This last, of course, is everyday apparent in psychiatric practice and social work care.

Little wonder, then, that narrative occupies an important place in the fields of palliative care and bereavement. This was borne in on me during my time as a carer, and reinforced when I came to chair meetings of the 'Users' Education Advisory Group' at St Christopher's Hospice. In the latter setting it was often personal experience, expressed in narrative, which enabled members of the group to contribute so well, yielding insights and understandings of where greater input might best be directed in helping patients and carers. During the course of the group's discussions it brought a sharp reality to the dilemmas and stresses they faced, frequently overriding logical analysis or academic dissection of needs and situations. Above all it served to underline the particular needs of the individual which can otherwise so easily become eclipsed.

I have therefore found this compilation of chapters, written by those well versed in end-of-life care, of unusual interest and value. It is rewarding to see how studies of narrative and storytelling can be utilized as a vehicle for scientific exploration and employed in various fields of research. To this end the underlying concepts are carefully defined and clarified, and the techniques of narrative interviewing dissected and analysed. It is gratifying also to read of the benefits that can accrue to patients by the skilful use of narrative and storytelling in therapy. In the splendid and moving chapter on 'Bereavement, children and families', it becomes apparent that in working with children such activities come into their own as a means of carrying matters forward and serving as an essential aid to remediation. Elsewhere we find evidence of the value of activities such as creative writing in putting patients in touch with their feelings and liberating them to express their innermost personal thoughts.

There is room only to mention a few of the other striking themes embodied in the various presentations. For example, we see how attention to narrative accounts can highlight the diverse meanings attributed by patients to their symptoms, particularly to the symptom of pain, and how differences in background, ethnicity, and culture can shape these attributions. Without a grasp of such issues the approach of attending professionals can miss much of the richness in the picture and come to overlook ways of intervening helpfully. Moreover narrative, as an expression of deeply personal feelings, lends an important counterbalance to the increasing technology of modern medicine in reinstating such matters as empathy and understanding in patient care.

In the chapter dealing with the role of patients and carers there are two remarkable stories which illustrate the importance, if it was ever in doubt, of listening attentively to the 'consumer's' point of view (Chapter 8). This indeed was at the heart of Cicely Saunders' journey towards establishing her model of hospice care. The chapter on 'Spirituality and the search for meaning' will open new horizons and understandings to many and expand them for all of us. It addresses a host of issues which too readily run the risk of being eclipsed when dealing with patients during crises in their lives. After reading it one feels acutely the barrenness of many of the interactions and experiences encountered during the course of busy general hospital care.

Altogether the message of this book becomes clear – in addition to the several functions of narrative mentioned in the opening paragraph, we discover a host of other applications which we might not have suspected. Though seeming at first glance to be modest and everyday activities, narrative and storytelling are clearly replete with promise in the field of palliative care. They serve to fill essential gaps, and they occupy a key role in placing the individual at the centre of the picture. In refining the way forward for end-of-life care, and in helping with bereavement, it can be argued that in many ways this is what matters most of all.

Index

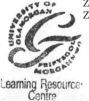

Learning Resource
Centre